J. Langdon Down

On Some of the Mental Affections of Childhood and Youth

Being the Lettsomian lectures delivered before the Medical society of London in

1887, together with other papers

J. Langdon Down

On Some of the Mental Affections of Childhood and Youth
Being the Lettsomian lectures delivered before the Medical society of London in 1887, together with other papers

ISBN/EAN: 9783337369965

Printed in Europe, USA, Canada, Australia, Japan

Cover: Foto ©Thomas Meinert / pixelio.de

More available books at **www.hansebooks.com**

ON SOME OF THE

MENTAL AFFECTIONS

OF

CHILDHOOD AND YOUTH

BEING

THE LETTSOMIAN LECTURES

DELIVERED BEFORE THE MEDICAL SOCIETY OF LONDON
IN 1887

TOGETHER WITH OTHER PAPERS

BY

J. LANGDON DOWN, M.D.Lond.

FELLOW OF THE ROYAL COLLEGE OF PHYSICIANS OF LONDON; SENIOR PHYSICIAN TO, AND
LECTURER ON CLINICAL MEDICINE AT, THE LONDON HOSPITAL; FORMERLY LECTURER
ON MEDICINE, MATERIA MEDICA, AND COMPARATIVE ANATOMY AT THE LONDON
HOSPITAL; AND PHYSICIAN TO THE EARLSWOOD ASYLUM

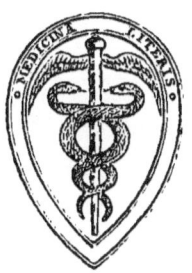

LONDON
J. & A. CHURCHILL
11, NEW BURLINGTON STREET
1887

PREFACE

When the Medical Society of London honoured me with the request to publish these Lectures, I felt, in complying with the wish so kindly expressed, that I should add to the value of the contribution by reprinting fugitive papers relating to the same subject, to some of which I have referred in the Lectures themselves. These papers I have printed in chronological order as the most convenient form.

J. LANGDON DOWN.

81, Harley Street, W.;
May, 1887.

CONTENTS

MENTAL AFFECTIONS OF CHILDHOOD AND YOUTH.

LECTURE I.

History of the Subject.—Nomenclature.—Ethnic Classification. — Etiological Classification. — Physical Characteristics.—Intellectual Characteristics   PAGES 1—42

LECTURE II.

Causes of Idiocy.—Accidental Origin.—Developmental Origin.—Congenital Origin.—Influence of Maternal Health; of Alcoholism; of Malignant Disease and Syphilis; of Neurotic or Phthisical Inheritance; of Trades and Professions; of Marriages of Consanguinity; of Illegitimacy; Idiocy from Deprivation of Senses; Cretinism; Influence of "Over-Education" of Women   .   .   .   43—90

LECTURE III.

Infantile Mania.—Melancholia and Delusions.—Moral Insanity.—"Idiots Savants."—Variations in the Mental Condition.—Epilepsy and Catalepsy.—Physical Deformities.—Associated Diseases.—Rate of Growth.—Diagnosis of Idiocy.—" Backward Children."—Deferred or Absent Speech.—Morbid Anatomy.—Treatment of Feeble-mindedness   91—142

CONTENTS.

	PAGES
Account of a Case in which the Corpus Callosum and Fornix were imperfectly formed and the Septum Lucidum and Commissura were Absent	143—153
On the Condition of the Mouth in Idiocy	154—166
On Polysarcia and its Treatment	167—180
An Account of a Second Case in which the Corpus Callosum was defective	181—184
Marriages of Consanguinity in relation to Degeneration of Race	185—209
Observations on an Ethnic Classification of Idiots	210—217
On Idiocy and its Relation to Tuberculosis	218—230
A Case of Asymmetrically Developed Brain	231—235
A Case of Microcephalic Skull	236—238
A Case of Microcephalic Skull	239—241
A Case of Arrested Development	242—244
A Case of Paralysis with apparent Muscular Hypertrophy	245—256
A Case of Pseudo-hypertrophic Paralysis	257—267
On the Relation of the Teeth and Mouth to Mental Development	268—288
The Obstetrical Aspects of Idiocy	289—307

MENTAL AFFECTIONS OF CHILDHOOD AND YOUTH.

LECTURE I.

History of the Subject.—Nomenclature.—Ethnic Classification.—Etiological Classification.—Physical Characteristics.—Intellectual Characteristics.

WHEN you, sir, and your colleagues on the Council of the Medical Society of London, did me the honour to request me to deliver the Lettsomian Lectures on Medicine for this year, I bethought myself that mental deviations in childhood and youth had never been the subject of a disquisition from this chair, and that probably a period of nearly thirty years spent among children with various phases of mental affection might entitle me to bring before the members of this Society material which, from the nature of the subject, can only be accumulated by a few.

There is not much to be found on this subject in the early records of medicine. Children who were afflicted by mental alienation or mental incapacity of any kind were placed in the category of idiots and regarded as beyond the pale of help. Formerly no attempt was made to ameliorate their condition, and a Spartan-like policy was rife, which troubled itself only with the survival of the fittest. It has been reserved for the medicine of modern times to occupy itself about the waifs of humanity who come under the category of the feeble in mind. The earliest attempts at the education of idiots took place in France some years since, but they were at first isolated efforts under the direction of M. Séguin at the Bicêtre. It was, however, in 1842 that attention was more particularly directed to the subject by the establishment of a school on the Abendberg, in Switzerland, which was opened by Dr. Guggenbühl, who entered on his work with true enthusiasm,—an enthusiasm which one regrets was quenched by the flattery of English drawing-rooms. I shall never forget the feelings of disappointment and chagrin when, on reaching the summit of the Abendberg, which I had mounted as a pilgrim to a shrine, I found the pupils in a state of physical and mental neglect while the patron saint was being enervated by the Capua-like influence of the West

End of London. Fortunately for the pupils the Commune stepped in and closed what had become a parody on philanthropic effort.

About the same time M. Saegert, at Berlin, who had been engaged in the instruction of deaf mutes, extended his efforts for the benefit of a class whose mutism was not the outcome of deafness. His school is still carried on with much skill in the neighbourhood of Berlin, but with the immense disadvantage of being located in, and associated with, a large lunatic asylum. On a recent visit which I paid it I found excellent work was being done there although handicapped by the association to which I have referred. It was in the year 1846 that a general movement took place in efforts for ameliorating this afflicted class. Germany took the lead by the establishment of a school at Leipzig. Discussions in the periodical press were initiated by Mrs. Plumbe, of London, whose personal interest in the matter forced the subject on the attention of such philanthropists as Dr. Conolly and Dr. Andrew Reed. Synchronously, public attention was being given to the subject in the United States of America, where, while politicians were delaying action in the matter, the private enterprise of the late Dr. Wilbur brought it to a practical issue. England meanwhile commenced the work by the establishment of a small school at Bath. It was not, however, till 1847 that the great effort was made which resulted in starting a small institution at Highgate in 1848 and subsequently another at Colchester. These grew into the large institution at Earlswood, of which in 1858, at the mingling of the inmates from these homes at Highgate and Colchester, I undertook the superintendence. In recent years other institutions have been created both in England, Ireland, Scotland, the United States, and on the Continent of Europe. Schools have been established at Darenth for the feeble-minded paupers of London. One hopes that the time may not be far distant when suitable provision may lie within the reach of the afflicted poor who live beyond the metropolitan area.

It is not uncommon to class all cases of mental lesion occurring in the young under the category of idiocy, or to speak of those afflicted with the graver forms of the malady as idiots, while the subjects of the milder or less grave manifestations are called imbeciles. This nomenclature is open to grave objection. The term imbecile is very often applied to that class of mental infirmity which is the outcome of deteriorating organic causes, often senile. Men or women who may have been in their time capable citizens become the subjects of senile changes of nutrition and lapse into a condition of childishness. It is people of this class who are rightly termed imbeciles, and to whom in my opinion the designation should be thoroughly restricted. I know of no defining limitation between so-called idiocy and so-called imbecility. The gradations of mental incapacity are as numerous and delicate as are those of mental capacity among those who are doing the world's work. The division, therefore, into imbeciles and idiots is thoroughly wrong and misleading. I have no great liking for the term idiot. It is so frequently a name of reproach. Moreover, in most cases it does not fairly represent the conditions which exist. The word idiot means "solitary," and the typical idiot knows nothing, sees nothing, does nothing, and this typical idiot is scarcely ever met with except in anencephalous monsters. This objection to the term idiot is not a mere sentimental one on my part. No one likes the name, and no mother will admit that her child deserves the title. The constant introduction of a case from medical men is, "I send you a little child for your opinion, but it is not an idiot;" or the mother brings her child to one, saying, "I have come to consult you about my boy, but he is not an idiot." This is the regular formula. A great impediment is thereby introduced to the early appreciation of the lesion and to its early treatment. The term idiot might be advantageously replaced by that of feeble-minded, idiocy being in fact mental feebleness depending on malnutrition or disease of the nervous centres taking place anterior to birth or during the developmental years of childhood and youth. Idiocy is therefore readily differentiated from other forms of mental alienation. The term imbecile should be applied to the cases of dementia which crowd our lunatic asylums and who are in an entirely different category from the feeble-minded; they are gradually deteriorating in physical, mental, and moral condition; they are in the position of spendthrifts who have dissipated their fortune, while idiots for the most part have never entered on a fortune to dissipate.

Some years since I was struck by the remarkable resemblance of feeble-minded children to the various ethnic types of the human family, and showed, in a paper which I contributed to the 'London Hospital Reports' in 1866, in how many instances one could refer them to one or other of the ethnological families. I have had under my care typical examples of the negroid family, with characteristic malar bones, the prominent eyes, the puffy lips and retreating chin. They have had the woolly hair, although not black, nor has the skin acquired pigmentary deposit. They have been examples of white negroes, but of European descent. Several, again, have arranged themselves around the Malay variety, with soft, black, curly hair, prominent upper jaws and capacious mouths, types of the South Sea Islands. I have also met with a few instances of the North American Indian type, with shortened forehead, prominent cheeks, deep-set eyes and slightly apish nose. A considerable number range themselves under the Mongolian type. More than 10 per cent. of congenital, feeble-minded children are typical Mongols. They present characteristics so marked that when the members of this type are placed in proximity it is difficult to believe that they are not brothers and sisters. In fact their resemblance is infinitely greater to one another than to the members of their own families. They rarely have black hair, as in the real Mongol, but it is of a brownish colour, straight and sparse. The face is flat and broad and destitute of prominence. The cheeks are roundish and widened laterally. The eyes are obliquely placed and the internal canthi more than normally separated. The palpebral fissure is very narrow, the forehead is wrinkled transversely from the constant use of the occipito-frontalis muscle in opening the eyes. The lips are large and thick, with transverse fissures. The tongue is long and thick and very rugous. The nose is small. The skin has a tawny colour, and is deficient in elasticity, giving on the hands the appearance of being larger than is necessary. The ethnic classification of idiocy which I indicated is of extreme interest philosophically as well as of value practically. Philosophically because it throws light on a question which very much agitated public opinion about the time of the American Civil War. The work of Nott and Gliddon laboured to prove that the various ethnic families were distinct species, and a strong argument was based on this to justify a certain domestic institution. If, however, it can be shown that from some deteriorating influence the children of Caucasian parents can be removed into another ethnic type, it is a strong corroborative argument that the difference is a variable and not a specific one. The classification is also a practical one. We are able to say, with the greatest possible certainty, that the members of these ethnic types date the origin of their mental feebleness to congenital causes.

It is often of great importance to determine the question as to whether the affliction has had an accidental beginning. The medical attendant may be charged with malpraxis. The nurse may be suspected of having allowed the infant to fall or of having drugged it with opiates. The being able to refer the child to an ethnic type other than Caucasian settles beyond question that the cause of the malady, whatever it may be, was antecedent to birth. Again and again has this process of reasoning come to my assistance in determining questions of the gravest possible import, and enabled me to assure anxious friends that innocent people have been unjustly blamed. Not only so, by a recognition of type we are able to determine the physical as well as mental and moral characteristics of the child in a way which astonishes the mother, who finds one is able to anticipate all she has to relate. This is especially the case with the Mongolian type, the numerous instances of which coming under one's notice enables one to become familiar with its leading characteristics. These children have always great power of imitation and become extremely good mimics. Several patients who have been under my care have been wont to convert their pillow-slips into surplices and to imitate, in tone and gesture, the clergyman or chaplain they have recently heard. Their power of imitation is moreover not limited to things clerical. I have known a ventriloquist to be convulsed with laughter between the first and second parts of his entertainment on seeing a Mongolian patient mount the platform, and hearing him grotesquely imitate the performance with which the audience had been entertained. They have a strong sense of the ridiculous; this is indicated by their humorous remarks and the laughter with which they hail accidental falls, even of those to whom they are most attached. Another feature is their great obstinacy,—they can only be guided by consummate tact. No amount of coercion will induce them to do that which they have made up their minds not to do. Sometimes they initiate a struggle for mastery, and the day previous will determine what they will or will not do on the next day. Often they will talk to themselves, and they may be heard rehearsing the disputes which they think will be the feature of the following day. They in fact, go through a play in which the patient, doctor, governess, and nurses are the *dramatis personæ*,—a play in which the patient is represented as defying and contravening the wishes of those in authority. Whether it be the question of going to church, to school, or for a walk, discretion will often be the better part of valour, by not giving orders which will run counter to the intended disobedience, and thus maintaining the appearance of authority while being virtually beaten. They are always amiable both to their companions and to animals. They are not passionate nor strongly affectionate. They are usually able to be taught to speak; the speech, however, is somewhat thick and indistinct, and destitute of musical cadence. The co-ordinating faculty is abnormal, but may be greatly improved by training. The circulation is usually feeble, and whatever advance is made intellectually in the summer some amount of retrogression may be expected in the winter. They undergo, in fact, a species of hibernation; not only are they prone to chilblains and frost-bite, they are but little tolerant of excessive heat, and proximity to a fire which to many would be only agreeable would, to patients of this class, be attended by serious blistering of the legs, even when protected by stockings or other articles of clothing. The resemblance to one another is so great in members of this family, both in their physical, moral, and intellectual natures, that the probability was forced on one that there was some unity of cause for their malady. Further investigation pointed out that phthisis was very frequently met with in the history of their progenitors. It is noticeable also that these children have not a long career, very few reaching adult life, being prone to succumb to serious illness or to become phthisical like their ancestors. Their crania have a marked similarity, they are all brachycephalic and the posterior part is ill-developed.

Latterly I have been accustomed to adopt a classification based on the etiology of the cases. This is valuable from its practical bearing, and because it brings into prominence a class which was formerly not considered, or at all events had not the attention given to it which it merited.

It was very early presented to my notice that a large number of feeble-minded children were capable of being referred to one or other of two great groups—the one where there was a complete history of the congenital origin of the malady, with the physical proofs, which I shall presently refer to, and the other where it was no less clear that the asseverations of the mother that her child was born with ordinary intelligence was quite correct, but that some accident or some extension of disease equivalent to an accident had wrought on the cerebral centres disastrous changes, interfering with intellectual manifestations. Parents always prefer to refer the case to a post-uterine or non-congenital origin, partly because they think it frees them from the suspicion of hereditary influence, and partly from a notion that the child is more likely to be restored to its pristine state. We have these two well-defined classes: (1) The congenital, and (2) the accidental. On investigating, however, a large number of cases I became familiar with many instances which it was impossible to include in either of these categories. There was no history of accident nor of any illness akin to accident; the examination, however thorough, revealed nothing which would warrant the opinion that the origin was accidental. There was, moreover, in these cases, no reason to regard them as congenital. On the contrary, all the historical evidence, as well as all the physical evidence, positively refuted any such idea.

Under what head, therefore, were they to be placed? I found that the history was somewhat of the following. Their early months of babyhood were perfectly uneventful; there had been nothing to cause the slightest anxiety; intelligence had dawned in the accustomed way, when, first dentition proceeding, a change had come over the aspect of the child. Its look had lost its wonted brightness; it took less notice of those around it; many of its movements became rhythmical and automatic, and with or without convulsions there was a cessation of the increasing intelligence which had marked its early career; anxiety was felt on account of the deferred speech, still more from the lessened responsiveness to all the endearments of its friends. In others the crisis at first dentition is not so marked. Speech may be a little deferred, but it comes, and with it more mental power; at second dentition, however, they are prone to crises in which the intelligence becomes altered, they have night terrors, and not unfrequently loss of speech. I have had many examples of children who had spoken well and with understanding, but who lost speech at the period of second dentition, and had also a suspension of mental growth.

I have now under my observation a boy who, except that he was a little backward in speaking, not talking till he was two years of age, attracted no particular attention during the first six years of his life. During the period of second dentition, without any fit or convulsion, he suddenly lost speech. He heard everything that was said, but never replied to a question. He would caress and coax, but never asked for what he wanted. It was not a case of aphonia; he appeared to have no power to convert ideas into words. He would cry peevishly if there was something he wanted that he could not have. This condition of things continued for eighteen months, when, suspecting masturbation, he was circumcised by Mr. Heath. Gradually, after two years' absence, speech returned. He had to be taught anew, first the names of objects, and then to build up sentences until, at the end of six months, my notebook says, " Speaks several sentences voluntarily." However, he afterwards always spoke of himself in the third person. He is now passing through the evolutionary period of puberty without any recurrence of the loss of speech faculty, but he has never regained active mental power. There is reason to regard it as a case of developmental feeble-mindedness resulting from illness of his mother at the seventh month of pregnancy.

I have had under my care two brothers who had spoken with discrimination and understood well two languages, but who both lost speech at the period of second dentition. As the elder one approached that period, gradually, without any paroxysmal event, he lost speech, and when the younger one arrived at the same age, gradually, but entirely, did he lose speech also. It may be, however, that the periods of first and second dentition are passed harmlessly and the breakdown is reserved for the time of puberty. Many at this time become suspicious and reserved, some become hyper-conscientious, are always practising a process of introspection, are disturbed in their mind lest they should not have rightly stated any circumstance, or, if they have correctly stated it, whether they have put the facts in such a way as to have produced the right impression; many become epileptic, with rapid declension of intellectual power. These cases have usually characteristic crania; they are dolichocephalic and are prow-shaped anteriorly,—the line corresponding to the medio-frontal suture being a prominent ridge. There is reason to believe that in these cases there has been an arrest of the synostosis of the medio-frontal suture which should have taken place during intra-uterine life, so that the lateral pressure on the separated frontal bones determines, when the deferred ossification takes place, a prominence where there should have been a plane or slightly concave surface between the frontal eminences. In the great bulk of these cases well-marked evidence can be obtained of some disturbing cause towards the later months of pregnancy, which has led to this condition; and although the deferred synostosis and its consequent deformity is of no consequence, it is reasonable to believe that the same cause which arrested the bony union has also arrested the development of the cerebral centres and rendered them more unstable. Certain it is that children with such a conformation are almost sure to break down at one or other of the developmental epochs. Their nervous system would appear to be equal to the requirements of growth but not of development. They form a class of cases which I have suggested should be called the " Developmental," as contradistinguished from the " Congenital " on the one hand, and the " Accidental " on the other. They are a very important class, because, forewarned, catastrophes may be avoided. They are the cases which break down by over-excitement in babyhood and by " over-pressure " in schools at second dentition and puberty. So frequent is the association of this condition of the cranium with neuroses that I have been accustomed for many years to point this out to my students at the London Hospital, and to show them that the prow-shaped skull is an outward and visible sign of an unstable nervous system, not of itself a cause, but indicating, like the seaweeds on the seashore, how far the tide has come. The members of this class do not give evidence of mental defect before their breakdown; they furnish, however, a number of those who become petulant, wayward vagrants from the elementary school, runaways from the public school, sometimes interesting and with flashes of precocious genius, they become the subjects of headache under continuous intellectual strain, a headache which, if not regarded, leads on infallibly to disastrous neuroses or developmental idiocy.

A large number of boys and girls come under my notice who are not feeble-minded, who have in a high degree the prow-shaped forehead, and who have their nervous system in such an unstable equilibrium that the least intellectual pressure at developmental epochs is attended by disastrous results. They are brought to me on account of severe frontal headache, or of wayward petulance, or incapacity for sustained mental exertion. I cannot better illustrate the kind of case which so frequently comes under my observation, and the serious character of which it is of the first importance early and clearly to recognise, than by quoting from the letter of the mother of one such patient. She says, "I have a boy eight and a half years old who is continually suffering with headache from temple to temple, and over the front half of head. He is a child of fine physique, capable, practical, clever, so far as the head permits of lessons, which means but a short amount and often missed altogether, for the same reason—'headache,'—apparently the picture of health, high spirits, active, bright, yet done up with so little. The child is not a rickety creature—more is the puzzle. We shall bring him to see you on Tuesday next, and I think it better to give you all particulars before our visit that you may form an opinion on the whole. In the Spring after a certain pressure of the usual morning work, he would turn grey, gasp for air, and, with windows all open, say he was choked. These attacks were frequent, and the sensations in the throat seemed to frighten him greatly. Lately I have heard less of this; now it seems 'head' affecting him 'all over' as he expresses it.

"Since then he has grown tall and much stronger, crickets fairly well, can handle any tool 'properly,' has good sense, good memory, a bad or rather tempestuous temper, quickly over, strong will, and ought to be a boy well to the front; but, alas for such hopes, there is ever a something cropping up which knocks it all over. Then fatigue, long journeys, lessons, and all is depression and pain, and a heavy dulness of power (never of intellect) which is heart-grieving to me. Writing tires him, yet he works his Latin sentences with ease aloud, only two a day. Two hours' work has become half an hour, sometimes lately five minutes. He remains still over-full of life and go, at times, with no *real* strength, irritable, open, upright, self-willed, loving, *very true*, still *all wrong*, and why?"

When the boy presented himself to me he displayed a typical neurotic forehead, and there was a very complete history of severe emotional disturbance on the part of the mother between the sixth and seventh month of pregnancy. I counselled complete abstention from intellectual work during the remaining period of second dentition. It was very clear to my mind that any continued pressure would lead, through convulsions, to developmental idiocy.

Dr. West has pointed out how stammering never occurs among young children, and says, " I never knew a child stammer before the commencement of the second dentition." My own experience would lead me to confirm the observations of that distinguished physician, and I would further say that I have never met with a case of stammering at that period which did not bear evidence of its being a developmental neurosis, and that its origin could be traced back to a period anterior to birth, to an arrest of development which begat a proclivity to nervous breakdown. In these cases the approach of puberty is a period of grave anxiety. It is at that time that masturbation is so liable to lead to disastrous results, and that epilepsy is so prone to occur. The nervous system may have been stable through the developmental periods of first and second dentition and yet break down at the evolution of puberty, and there is much sagacity in Dr. West's observation: "It is usually with the evolution of the sexual system that hysteria shows itself, and with the pressure of life's cares that the mind is thrown off its balance, and then it is with regard to both that the ancestral taint first displays itself; so too, is it, I believe, to a great degree with the hereditary tendency to epilepsy." It is, I would venture to say, the influence of the neurotic mother on the embryo during the later months of development that begets the proclivity which is here referred to.

I have alluded already to a group which I have ventured to describe as "accidental." I wish thereby to refer to a class of cases which differ from the "developmental" in the date of the origin of their calamity. They are children who are born, or ready to be born, with all the potentiality of intelligence, but whose brain becomes damaged by traumatic lesions, by medications, or by inflammatory disease. There is this one character running through the class,—a character on which I wish to lay as great stress as I have on the prow-shaped cranium of the developmental class, viz. the absence of any of the physical aspects of feeble-mindedness. They are bright in their expression, often active in their movements, agile to a degree, mobile in their temperament, fearless as to danger, persevering in mischief, petulant to have their own way. Their language is one of gesture only; living in a world of their own they are regardless of the ordinary circumstances around them, and yield only to the counter-fascination of music.

These are the cases in which mothers entertain the strongest hope, and in which the doctor endorses the hope with confidence based on the pretty waywardness of the child. I cannot enforce too strongly grave caution in the prognosis which should be given in such cases; they are the most disappointing which one is called upon to treat. A period of nearly thirty years has enabled me to study not only the present but the future of such children, to make a forecast, based on experience as to results, and to correct the notions of sanguine hopefulness. So interesting are they in appearance that it is difficult to realise that they will not be perfectly responsive to training, and that speech will not be speedily gained. I know nothing more painful than the long motherly expectancy of speech; how, month after month, the hopes are kept at high tension, waiting for the prattle which never comes. How the self-contained and self-absorbed little one cares not to be entertained other than in his own dreamland, and by automatic movements of his fingers or rhythmical movements of his body. I cannot recommend too strongly that caution should be used in giving a hopeful prognosis concerning children of this class. They have well-formed heads, finely-textured skins, well-chiselled mouths, sparkling eyes, features when in repose leading one to augur only brightness and intelligence. Surely, it may be thought, the mind is ready to be developed from such a casket, and time only is required to ensure the thorough realisation of all one's wishes. Opinions based on such a theory will prove utterly fallacious. In these cases there is no outward sign of mental vacuity, for there has been nothing during the period of intra-uterine life to arrest the evolutionary stages, and stamp its impress on the bodily or facial formation. The cause of the mental deficiency has been something occurring during post-uterine life,—some catastrophe not inherent in the child, no hereditary taint to mar the beauty of his visage or the grace of his cranial contour; yet there is something more potent for evil than in the case of many a malformed face and many a distorted skull. He runs to you when called, but makes no response in words. He returns your kiss by a bite, and runs away with agile steps, rolling his head with a horizontal swaying motion, or with fingers in ears or at eyeballs producing distorted sounds or double vision, and as he goes, rushing to knock down objects in order to produce an unharmonious noise. They are cases with a vast amount of surplus nervous energy, and although much may be done by training to divert the energy into better channels, the improvement will be smaller than what may be obtained from apparently less promising children, because, as I have elsewhere said, there is more improvement to be obtained from an ill-developed than from a damaged brain.

The late Professor Griesinger, with whom I have frequently had opportunities of discussing this and kindred subjects, describes two varieties of idiots—the apathetic and the excited. The apathetic class he describes as awkward, clumsy, and disproportioned, with repulsive old-looking features. From their torpor and impassiveness they seem to be in a dreamy state. Their expression is either brooding and melancholy, or vacuous and indifferent. The excited or agitated class he describes as just as stupid as the other, but quick in movement and irritable, passing rapidly from one impression to another, and quite incapable of fixing anything on their minds. I have no doubt Griesinger had in view, in describing the latter class, some of the accidental cases whose manifestations I have been discussing. There is no attempt, however, in this classification to refer them to their cause, nor can I admit that the division is true to nature or practically useful.

Having thus discussed two of the great classes, the accidental and the developmental, there remains for me to describe the characteristics of the remaining one, viz. the congenital. This contains by far the largest number of subjects, and presents characters which are of great value in determining the origin and future of its members. They are less interesting in appearance but more amenable to training, other things being equal, than either of the other two classes, and especially than the members of the accidental class. The origin of their malady dates from earlier in intra-uterine life than does that of the members of the developmental class, and in many cases the proclivity resides in the germ-cell or sperm-cell, as the result of gradual degeneration. That being so, it is not surprising that members of this class should bear in their bodily formation marks of physical change. They for the most part have a tendency to fall under one or other of the ethnic groups which I referred to in the early part of this lecture. Some years since I gave great attention to this subject, and prepared much material for a paper on the physical aspects of idiocy. A great many descriptions had been written, by no means precise, on the intellectual condition of idiots, but none, so far as I know, on their physical attributes. It is now several years since that this city was excited by the trial before a Master in Lunacy of a young man whose ability to manage his affairs was doubted. The author of 'Ten Thousand a Year' presided at the trial. Experts on both sides gave evidence on the psychological condition. The late Lord Cairns (then Sir Hugh) was the advocate for the youth, and he argued strongly that the error had been fallen into of supposing this young man was feeble-minded because he had a high arched palate, and in other ways a deformed mouth, so that his defective utterances had given rise to the opinion that he was deficient in mental power. From the material I had collected I wrote a paper for the 'Lancet' to show that, granted any suspicion of defective mental power, the deformation of the mouth, with its vaulted palate, was the strongest corroborative proof, a proof too of the congenital origin of his condition. My paper was too late to enable the opposite side to call me, and it could only be made use of in the opposing counsel's final address. The jury supported the doctrine of the liberty of the subject, and the poor congenital imbecile was allowed to go his own way to destruction, with the result of becoming speedily bankrupt in fortune, ruined in health, and a scandal to an honoured ancestral name.

Still more recently, a youth on coming of age sought to obtain possession of his property.

There was strong evidence brought as to his conduct being incompatible with mental capacity, and the physical deviations were confirmatory of the congenital character of the feeble-mindedness. The jury, however, decided by a small majority that he was capable of managing his own affairs, although they were equally divided as to his mental soundness. Within forty-eight hours he was in prison for gross criminal conduct, and he speedily terminated a career of infamy from want of legal protection, which the poor feeble-minded youth could not give to himself. In the cases I am describing the cranium is usually smaller than normal, dolichocephalic in many but brachycephalic in the Mongolian type. Occasionally the head is scaphocephalic, the line of the sagittal suture giving a keel-like feature to what resembles an inverted boat. A very common character is a rapid shelving from the vertex posteriorly, corresponding to what is so frequently to be noticed, an arrest of development of the occipital lobe of the cerebrum. Not unfrequently the cranium is extremely small, reverting to the Aztec type. These examples of extreme microcephalism have been attributed by Virchow to premature synostosis of the cranial sutures. I have found, however, that in some of the most marked members of the microcephalic group the sutures are well marked and every indication that the cranium had adapted itself to the cerebrum rather than that the cerebral mass had been dominated by the cranium. They are cases in which the brain and bony covering are both in miniature, the arrest having had an early intra-uterine date. It would be a grave error to imagine that there is an inverse relation between the size of the cranium and the intellectual capabilities of its possessor. I have known children with the most complete Aztec-like heads susceptible of some amount of education; they have been taught to talk, to discriminate, to take a real pleasure in the world around them, appreciate the jokes in a dramatic entertainment, and play intelligently with toys. I have under my care now one who has been taught to speak with discrimination, to say the conventional thing, to play on the piano simple airs, to read story books with enjoyment, and to have a practical appreciation of right and wrong. They are usually mobile in temperament, sometimes very active physically, and always tractable, amiable, and appreciative of kindness. They illustrate the fact that there is such a thing as quality in brain-matter as well as quantity, and that the relative intelligence among feeble-minded children cannot be estimated simply by the tape and calipers. Macrocephalic crania are not unfrequently met with, some being due to hydrocephalus, and others to an increase of the neuroglia of the cerebral mass. I have had patients under my care whose brains were within an ounce of the weight of that of Cuvier, who, nevertheless, were slow in their movements and slower in thought, and were perfect contrasts in intellectual sluggishness to the volatile microcephalic Aztecs with brains only one fourth the weight. An inspection in these cases revealed the fact that the cineritious portion was pale and that the increased weight was due to the increase of the white substance, and especially of its connective-tissue elements. Another deformation met with in congenital feeble-mindedness is a marked asymmetricality of the two sides of the cranium. There is also in many an increase of the facial development as compared with the cranial. The ears are implanted farther back relatively than in normal heads. The eyes have their canthi too closely approximated in the dolichocephalic cases and too widely separated in the brachycephalic. The palpebral fissures are often narrow and obliquely placed, and the forehead is, not unfrequently, corrugated in consequence of the employment of the occipito-frontalis muscle to raise the lid. At the inner canthi the integument often forms semilunar folds as if the skin were too scanty, which I have proposed to call epi-canthic folds. These are met with in people who are not feeble-minded, but they are more frequent in the latter and are, I believe, signs of degeneracy.

I have already referred to, and have elsewhere described in detail, the deformations of the mouth, which I regard as very important in the diagnosis of congenital idiocy. These views have been very generally adopted since I brought them under the notice of the profession. They have, however, been taken exception to in two different quarters and for different reasons. Dr. Kingsley, a distinguished dentist of New York, did me the honour to say that he had come to England mainly to discuss with me the question and to see my cases. It was evident to me that he had not had an opportunity of studying the same kind of cases, and he stated that he had met with the palates I have described in people not feeble-minded. I am not the less convinced that they are signs of degeneracy which, sooner or later, culminate in feeble-mindedness in the offspring, unless intermixed with a stronger strain. This view was confirmed by many members of the Odontological Society of London when I brought the subject before them. Mr. Keeling said "he had been induced to attend that meeting by the announcement of the paper to be read by Dr. Langdon Down. He had understood Dr. Down to ask for information respecting the gradual degeneration which might have taken place in the successive generations of the parents of imbecile children. He was in a position to afford such information. He knew the grandfather and mother of an imbecile child (the latter, he had reason to know, had been under the care of Dr. Down), and if the discussion were postponed he should be happy to produce the models of the mouths of the grandfather and the mother, and, perhaps, of the imbecile child's mouth also; and the models would show that a very marked and gradual deterioration of the palates and teeth had taken place in the mouths of the individuals referred to, from the grandfather to the imbecile child." Mr. Oakley Coles said that he "for some two years past had experimented upon the anatomy and physiology of the palate, and seemed to have been working side by side with Dr. Down. His results to a great extent confirmed those of that gentleman." The late Mr. Sercombe said, " Dr. Down's remarks about the high vaulted palate and lunacy being commonly associated had much struck him, and brought to his mind the conditions of one of the oldest families in the realm, who were patients of his, in whom every branch of the family had remarkably high V-shaped palates, and at least two members of the family had been in confinement." The President of the Odontological Society, the late Mr. Mummery, said "that he had occasionally noticed, in cases where the mental power was deficient, the front teeth were not on the same plane as the molars," an observation I am able to confirm. I am the more desirous of placing these opinions of members of the dental profession on record here because Dr. Kingsley, since his return to America, has read a paper "On the Development of the Teeth" before the Odontological Society of New York in which he reopens the question and makes statements which are not in harmony with my own experience. He says, "In meditating some time since upon the subject I came to the conclusion that, if my deductions were correct, I should find proof of it in an examination of sluggish or feeble intellect, and at that time I wrote this sentence: 'In an examination of idiots we shall be likely to find capacious jaws and teeth not crowded.' If a precocious or stimulated brain in infancy urges on and crowds the dental organs in advance of the growth of the jaws, then a brain of low calibre or power will be likely to have associated with it a retarded dentition, but with abundance of room. After this conclusion of my own," he says, "I came across a paper by Dr. Langdon Down. Dr. Down's statements, founded upon his observations of nearly a thousand feeble-minded patients, were so astounding, and so at variance with my theory, that the picture which I had painted seemed to vanish like a vision." Dr.

Kingsley, however, visited an asylum for idiots upon Rundall's Island in America, numbering about two hundred, and did not see a single pronounced case of v-shaped dental arch. On visiting my patients he says that "there was no mistaking the fact that there was a larger percentage of the kind of deformities which Dr. Down had described than I had found in any other collection of feeble-minded." Dr. Kingsley attributes the exceptional condition of the patients to their being members of the higher orders of society, but the fact is that my first observations were made on poorer children at Earlswood.

An able physician in England, Dr. T. Claye Shaw, has tried to show that there are many idiots with well-formed mouths and palates, and with this I agree if he includes accidental and developmental cases. My contest is that they are typical of the congenital class, and one value attaching to these observations is that they often afford a means of differentiating the latter from the two former classes. Dr. Bourneville, of Paris, has carried on investigations on the same subject in France, and in a memoir has generally confirmed my views. Dr. Ireland, in his treatise of 'Idiocy and Imbecility,' says, "Dr. T. Claye Shaw took the trouble to write a paper to prove that a highly arched palate is not a sign of the existence of idiocy and imbecility; that a palatal investigation cannot afford a clue to the mental faculties. Dr. T. Claye Shaw's paper illustrates the confusion of mind one must fall into who studies the physical aspects of idiocy, while he persists in regarding it as a class incapable of further subdivision."

The feeble-minded have a tendency to become stout, with great development of adipose tissue; an example of this I related in the 'London Hospital Reports' with the results of medication and diet.

Common sensation is generally much less acute than in ordinary persons. Pain is borne with wonderful callousness. It is not uncommon for children of this class to allow a thecal abscess to be opened with a scalpel without a grimace or without uttering a word. The same thing also applies to the extraction of teeth. This is quite in harmony with what may be expected; the hyper-sensitiveness of the cultured gentleman, as compared with the untutored ploughman, is matter of every-day observation, well illustrated in the case of the great Sir Robert Peel, whose sensitiveness cost him his life. Special sensation is also obtuse. Hearing is generally less acute, and this is often an important element in cases of delayed speech. We all know that absence of speech is often the outcome of complete deafness, but it is not sufficiently recognised that a very slight congenital defect of hearing, is sufficient to cause deferred and defective speech.

Lesions of sight are very frequent. Congenital cataract is very commonly associated with congenital feeble-mindedness. Several cases have also come under my notice of blindness the result of arrested development of the globe. Strabismus is very common, and nystagmus, though less common, is not infrequent. Myopia, but especially hypermetropia, is a frequent accompaniment of congenital mental lesions. Colour-blindness is occasionally met with, but it is difficult to say in how many cases it is from a want of mental power. The sense of smell is ill-developed in a great many and that of taste keeps company therewith. The most nauseous medicines are taken without question, and in fact with many its administration is regarded as a mark of attention and appreciated accordingly.

The muscular system is weak. Not only are physical efforts feeble, there is no power of sustained endurance. Co-ordination is defective and finely adjusted movements are exceptional. There is a great tendency to automatism and rhythmical actions. Salaams, horizontal swayings, and rotations of the head and body are often met with. The lack of muscular power makes itself painfully manifest in a number of instances by the postponement of walking or even of standing. This is a symptom which brings children of this class under the notice of the physician or surgeon. The mother magnifies all the little manifestions of intelligence, but she cannot understand why the child does not walk. There may be no spastic rigidity, no contractures, and yet the little legs are powerless; they would seem to be unable to obey the behests of the will even were there any will exercising its proper domain. In the large number of notes which I possess of congenital feeble-minded children, walking delayed to the third or fourth year is a very common occurrence. Imperfect prehension with the upper extremities is also a frequent characteristic, and often the vertical position is rendered impossible by virtue of muscular weakness long after children of a similar age are running about.

There is still one important character with children of this class, which is a great cause of anxiety, viz. postponed or absent speech. I have, in describing the accidental forms of feeble-mindedness, referred to speech as a faculty which is frequently absent, and in the "developmental" class as a faculty which, having been once possessed, sometimes vanishes at special epochs.

In the class we are now considering delayed speech is universal, permanent absence less common. The lesion of speech in these cases is the outcome of several factors. The form of the mouth is, as I have shown, often abnormal. The high, narrow-vaulted palate presents a formidable difficulty; this is apt to be intensified by the ill-development of the lower jaw, the horizontal ramus forming too obtuse an angle with the ascending ramus, so that labials are expressed with difficulty. In addition to this the tongue is large, flabby, and defective in its muscular movements, and these are ill-co-ordinated. Again, the congenital defective hearing I have referred to is often another factor. Still further, there is too frequently the potent cause of having no power to convert ideas into words, and, alas, the still more potent one of having no ideas to communicate.

I have thus, in the limited time at my disposal, endeavoured to bring before you the prominent features of what I regard as the three great natural divisions of the sufferers from a grave calamity. Some of the causes which have produced it will occupy our time at our next meeting.

LECTURE II.

Causes of Idiocy.—Accidental Origin.—Developmental Origin. —Congenital Origin.—Influence of Maternal Health; of Alcoholism; of Malignant Disease and Syphilis; of Neurotic or Phthisical Inheritance; of Trades and Professions; of Marriages of Consanguinity; of Illegitimacy; Idiocy from Deprivation of Senses; Cretinism; Influence of "Over-Education" of Women.

THE causes of idiocy or feeble-mindedness will always attract a good deal of attention, and will doubtless, as heretofore, lead to much speculative opinion. It will be obvious from the classification on which I have insisted that the causes vary in their nature and their date, in the three great divisions to which I have referred. In the "accidental" variety there is usually not much difficulty in arriving at the cause. The history, as a rule, elucidates the matter. Some are from injury received at birth by necessary instrumental interference, but it is very remarkable how few are sacrificed from this cause. Many years ago, when I was assistant to the late Dr. Ramsbotham, I remember his telling me that the cases were very few in which he could trace any cerebral lesion as resulting from the employment of the forceps, and he must have known many instances where the forceps, and especially the long forceps, had been applied less dexterously than they would have been by his marvellously accomplished hands. During the later years of Dr. Ramsbotham's life I took great pains to investigate the subject, and my results were greatly in accord with his assertion.

I found that among the great number of feeble-minded children about whom I could get thoroughly reliable accounts, in only 3 per cent., including members of the three great classes, had the forceps or any other instrument been employed. It is probable, therefore, that in 9 per cent. of purely accidental cases instrumental interference might have been the principal factor. Far more important, however, in the production of accidental cases, is the prolonged transmission of the child in the maternal passages. In the preparation of a paper for the Obstetrical Society of London I called attention to the fact that in so large a proportion as 20 per cent. of all idiots whose history I had investigated, there was an undoubted account of suspended animation at birth—a suspension requiring active efforts to bring about resuscitation. I believe that the members of our profession who have given attention to deformities among children could say how very frequently suspended animation at birth is associated with the contractures and other lesions which they are called upon to treat.

This cause is more frequently met with in first-born children, for the very obvious reason that the transit of the child is more likely to be delayed to a perilous extent by the smallness of the internal passages and the rigidity of the perinæum usually associated with a primiparous birth. Ergot of rye, when administered to the mother during the parturient hours, has been thought to be a cause of accidental idiocy, but the result of my inquiries has been to establish in my mind a verdict of " not proven." In many of the cases in which ergot has been employed, the very condition for which it was used, viz. delayed transit of the child, has been the cause of the evil rather than the agent which was intended to hasten the birth. Moreover, it is extremely difficult to obtain from the mother any information of what was or what was not administered during the period of her peril. The outcome of these remarks is, I think, to show that, independently of what concerns the safety of the mother, mental and physical evil to the child is more likely to be induced by prolonged pressure and a delayed use of instruments than by the early and adroit employment of agents likely to hasten the birth.

Insolation in infancy is certainly a cause of accidental idiocy. It has fallen to my lot to see a notable number of feeble-minded children who owe their disaster to sunstroke while making the passage of the Red Sea and Suez Canal *en route* from India, or from exposure in that country. I have at the present time under my care a very good example. There is every reason to regard the case as an accidental one, having reference to the history and the physical configuration of the child, while the mental decadence dates without question from the period when exposure was unavoidable.

The administration of opium by nurses to keep their charges quiet is often regarded by parents as a possible cause of their little one's defect. From the nature of the case it is very difficult to prove the administration of the drug, and even if that be proved, to associate it with the lesion. I am led to regard this as a very infrequent cause of accidental idiocy, inasmuch as the majority of the cases, where strong assertions have been made as to the furtive administration of the medicament, have in their persons indubitable evidence of the congenital nature of the malady, and, moreover, evidence usually that the cause must be traced far back in intra-uterine life. Much more tangible as a cause is morbid sexual erethism, too often induced by nurses who procure the quietness of their charge by means which, even if the mental health is not sacrificed, lead eventually to grave moral delinquencies. A not insignificant portion, however, break down, and mental hebetude becomes their lot. I would impress on you strongly my conviction that this evil has a very early significance, and the probability of the occurrence must always be kept in view.

Traumatic injury to the cranium from falls may be, and doubtless is, a cause of accidental idiocy. It is readily conceivable that injuries of this kind may prove harmful immediately by concussion or later on by secondary lesions of the brain and its membranes. I am persuaded, however, that it is not so common as a cursory consideration might lead one to believe. A large number of cases are referred by the mothers to falls or suspected falls, the objective evidence of which is entirely opposed to such a theory, cases in which the congenital nature of the affection is beyond dispute. Traumatic causes like opium drugging are, I am convinced, but rarely factors in the production of feeblemindedness.

Meningitis, on the other hand, very frequently leads to this variety of idiocy. A large number of cases of accidental idiocy have somewhat of this history. They have been born with undoubted intelligence; they have contracted scarlatina, measles, or smallpox; this has been followed by inflammation of the ear with extension to the membranes of the brain, or the otitis may be set up by catarrh, the inflammatory action extending from the outer to the middle ear or from the pharynx by means of the Eustachian tube. Whatever the origin death does not always take place, the little sufferer undergoes a perilous illness with violent convulsions, and, escaping with life, is not unfrequently left in a condition of mental feebleness. I have made many autopsies in which there was evidence of a long past inflammatory process and in which there was a probability that the anæmic condition of the cerebral convolutions had for a cause the constringing effect on the vessels, of organised lymph at the base of the brain.

Epileptiform convulsions, whether eclampsic or not, frequently cause accidental idiocy. These may be induced by peripheral irritation of any kind, and, as Dr. West has pointed out in his suggestive and elegant Lumleian lectures, " be the cause what it may by which the fit is first excited, a paroxysm of whooping-cough or the irritation of thread-worms,—something which would seem most temporary in its character and furthest removed from any abiding influence on the higher endowments of the nervous system, it yet leaves behind a mark, a stamp, a stain, not unlike what theologians tell us of the flaw which our first parents' sin has left upon our moral nature,—a predisposition in short to a great evil." It is, however, in the kind of idiocy which I have termed "developmental" that the results of epileptiform convulsions are the most manifest.

Hydrocephalus is also an occasional cause of accidental idiocy, more frequently, however, of the congenital variety. I have had under my care a few cases where the hydrocephalus became developed after birth and lessened or destroyed the intellectual faculties of the child.

Paralysis arising from cerebral hæmorrhage occurs as a cause of accidental as well as congenital idiocy. The amount of intellectual defect varies greatly, some cases are very amenable to instruction while others fail to respond to the efforts made for their benefit. In one case under my care the patient has been taught to play the violin fairly well, well enough to give him great pleasure, using the right hand instead of the left for fingering.

We now come to the causes of developmental idiocy, and I would first mention the maternal health during pregnancy, which is, I am convinced, a very potent factor in the production of that kind of idiocy which I have named "developmental," especially is it so if the deviation takes place during the sixth or seventh month.

The causes which, occurring early in the embryonic life of the child produce congenital, operating later produce developmental idiocy, by which I mean, as I explained in my first lecture, children born with intelligence but whose nervous and intellectual system breaks down at one or other of the developmental epochs.

The health deviations which lead up to this kind of idiocy are sickness, whether produced by the sea or other causes, uterine hæmorrhage, great emotional disturbance or grave febrile disease. The members of this class are very prone to eclampsia at first dentition, to epilepsy or chorea at second dentition, and to epilepsy or chorea, and moral deviations at the period of puberty. At any of these epochs there may be intellectual lesion varying in gravity with the nature of the malady. It is of the greatest importance that cases of this nature should be kept free from all exciting causes of nerve disturbance at the epochs referred to, and that intellectual pressure should be disallowed if we wish to avoid a greater catastrophe. With care in the directions referred to many of this class may escape the perils which want of caution will certainly induce. This is especially the class which breaks down from disturbing causes during the early period of puberty, and whose safety is only secured by frank exposition of the danger which results from moral delinquency.

The majority, however, of the children about whom opinion is desired falls properly under the head of the congenital class, and if it be asked, What is the cause of congenital idiocy? my reply is, that in a large number of cases one must seek for several factors. The more one inquires into the history of these cases the more one is convinced that the simple causation which has been referred to by several writers is fallacious, and that in one case to attribute it to intemperance only, in others to marriage of consanguinity, is to take a narrow view of the cause of the condition. I cannot but feel that the inquiry really becomes an inquiry into the pre-efficients or all that has gone to the making of idiocy. There can, I think, be no doubt that one of the great causes is heredity. It is impossible to devote much time to the elucidation of this subject without obtaining overwhelming proof of the transmissible nature of neurotic disease. If there are, as I am convinced, physical indications of the congenital trouble, there are also to be found in many of the progenitors indications of decadence. In the investigation into the antecedent history of 2000 cases, in 36 per cent. of the fathers I failed to get any history which could throw light upon the affliction, and the same failure occurred in 38 per cent. of the mothers, but in only 16 per cent. did I fail in obtaining a grave history of physical or psychical decadence from one or other of the progenitors. But even where there was no evidence of gross departure from a normal standard, one could not fail to notice frequently cranial and other signs of racial degeneration, such as narrow palates, rabbit mouths, bad foreheads and facial exaggerations. The causes of idiocy are not always operative in a single generation, and it is only by having the opportunity of examining into the physical conformation of parents and grandparents that one can see that idiocy in many cases is the culmination in the individual of a gradual degenerative process. Even with all the care

I have taken in the investigation I can only hope that my results are approximately correct. There is much difficulty in getting the information one needs on account of mistakes respecting the import of one's questions, and there are still further difficulties among those whose education would enable them to appreciate the inquiries made, owing to a desire on their part to keep in the background many points which would have a very important bearing on the problem. I have often found it useful to interrogate the parents separately, and have in this way obtained very useful data, each one in turn being not unwilling to supply all the facts which would appear to point to something in the opposite family as the potential cause of the affliction. I have endeavoured in such investigations to keep myself free from the bias of former statistics, especially those of the late Dr. Howe, of Massachusetts.

It had been a matter of speculation with me whether great disparity of age of the parents was not likely to be a cause, and strength was given to this supposition by a few remarkable cases which came under my observation—cases where the disparity was very great and where there was feeble-mindedness in the offspring. On making inquiries, however, over a large field, I was led to results which, though interesting, did not tend to confirm the speculative opinions I at first entertained. I found that the average age of the fathers of feeble-minded children at their birth was $35\frac{8}{12}$, and that of the mothers $31\frac{6}{12}$; a disparity of only $4\frac{2}{12}$ years. On looking about for some standard of comparison I met with Mr. Galton's statistics on the ages of the parents of men of scientific attainments at the period of their children's birth. Mr. Galton states that their father's average 36, and their mothers 30 years. With reference to the ages of the fathers in whose case we should naturally look for the potential cause there is a remarkable similarity, the advantage being on the side of the procreator of feeble-minded children to the extent of $\frac{4}{12}$ of a year, while there is less disparity of age among the parents of the feeble-minded than among the parents of men of prominent ability. The difference being six years in the case of Mr. Galton's selected men's parents as against $4\frac{2}{12}$ in the case of the parents of afflicted ones. It is clear, therefore, that disparity of age of the parents, although doubtless having an important influence on the wellbeing of the offspring, does not rank as an important factor in the production of idiocy.

It is worthy of remark that only 20 per cent. of the mothers gave birth to idiots at the age which Aristotle regarded as the most suitable one for a vigorous progeny, viz. between thirty and thirty-four. Whereas, according to Mr. Galton, no less than 34 per cent. of men of eminence are given birth to by their mothers at that age.

In a paper contributed to the Obstetrical Society of London I have indicated that there is a greater liability to idiocy among primiparous children; 24 per cent. of the 2000 idiots examined by me being first-born children. I found that seven was the average number of living children born to those parents who have had an idiot child, prolific child-bearing rather than the opposite appearing to be the characteristic of people begetting feeble-minded children. I ventured to suggest that the preponderance of idiocy in first-born children might be due to the exalted emotional life of the father and mother as well as to the increased difficulties of parturition, and to the attendant greater risk of suspended animation to which I have already referred. Curiously enough, while 24 per cent. of idiots generally are primiparæ no less than 40 per cent. of resuscitated idiots come under this category. I have long held and taught the opinion that suspension of animation must be regarded as one of the pre-efficients of idiocy.

I do not find that the production of twins is a very appreciable cause of idiocy. 2 per cent. only of my collection were twins, while, on the other hand, in 2 per cent. of my cases the mothers had given birth to twins who were not afflicted in any way.

I am aware that this opinion is rather different from that entertained by Dr. Arthur Mitchell, C.B. His statistics on the subject are somewhat different from mine. His observations were made in Scotland, and while I find that one in fifty idiots is one of twins, he found one in forty to come under this category. Having regard to the greater tendency to abnormal presentations, to the increased necessity for instrumental interference, and the greater liability to premature birth, I was prepared to expect a much larger number of idiots to have been twin children.

From what I have previously said it will be seen that I attach immense importance to the *emotional* life of the mother during the period of pregnancy, and I feel convinced it is one of the most potent of all the pre-efficients of idiocy. In 32 per cent. of my cases there was a well-ascertained history of great mental disturbance on the part of the mother at that time. My ever-to-be-revered teacher, the late Dr. W. B. Carpenter, relates how at the Siege of Landau in the year 1793, in addition to a violent cannonading, which kept the women in a constant state of alarm, the arsenal blew up with a terrific explosion, which few could bear with unshaken nerves. Out of 92 children born in that district within a few months afterwards 16 died at the time of birth, 33 languished from eight to ten months and then died, 8 became idiots and died before the age of five years, and 2 came into the world with numerous fractures of the bones of the limbs, probably caused by irregular uterine contractions. I can from my own experience refer to the number of cases of feeble-mindedness which were the outcome of the Siege of Lucknow, and in many others the result of sudden shocks from the receipt of distressing tidings of death or other calamities.

Another element in the etiology of idiocy is the *physical* health of the mother during the period of pregnancy. In 20 per cent. of my cases there was marked physical disturbance. In 4 per cent. of these there was a history of serious falls, falls from which uterine hæmorrhage followed; the other cases were those in which there was prolonged ill-health and in which *vomiting* was a prominent symptom. They were all such events or ailments as would be likely to interfere with the nutritive life of the embryo.

By far the most potent influence in the production of idiocy is the general physical and mental health of the progenitors. This I have already touched upon in speaking of heredity. One cannot fail to be struck by the nature of the stock from which such patients have sprung, and one has not far to seek for most potent causes. If, after a perusal of Mr. Galton's statistics of the antecedents of men of science, we compare the antecedents of my 2000 cases, the contrast is so great that all wonder at the production of mental feebleness vanishes. With fathers phthisical and irascible, with mothers feeble in judgment and so emotional that everything is a cause of fright, one is astonished that they should have procreated any sane child at all, and, indeed, in some cases the whole progeny of these parents is puny and feeble, failing to perform social duties. I find that in 16 per cent. of the cases there was insanity or marked feeble-mindedness on the father's side of the family, and in 15 per cent. there was the same condition on the mother's side. Severe emotional disturbance, bordering on insanity, occurred in 4 per cent. of the fathers, while a like affection in the mothers occurred in 13 per cent. These cases of emotional disturbance were very marked. Some of uncontrollable passion, ill-regulated grief, or morbid sentiment; others where clergymen had given up their cures through needless fear of stopping in the middle of their sermons; others, again, where ruin had been brought about by alienation of friends or ill-regulated lives.

I have found it very difficult to get at reliable statements with regard to the influence of alcoholic intemperance. There is not only a desire to conceal the fact, but there is evidently such an elastic gauge as to what constitutes intemperance that my numbers must be regarded as much within the truth. There was, however, avowed and notorious intemperance in 12 per cent. of the fathers and 2 per cent. of the mothers. I found, however, that the proportion varied extremely with the stratum of society from which my records were taken. In the members of the upper ranks in the social scale it was an insignificant factor, while when the inquiries related to the lower social class it became a factor of great importance, and in fact there appeared to be a gradually increasing percentage as the lowest stratum was reached.

I feel quite sure that drunkenness must be placed among the factors in the production of idiocy. I have had under my observation several families in which the majority of the children were mentally feeble, and the whole more or less fatuous, whose fathers were never *very* drunk yet never perfectly sober, and in these cases the chronic alcoholism had produced a condition of mental hebetude from the slow poisoning to which they were subjected.

Some of the cases are the result of slow deterioration of the father's mental and physical powers, others are the result of procreation having taken place during a debauch. I have elsewhere called attention to cases of idiocy resulting from well-authenticated instances, where procreation could only have occurred under such a condition. Such cases have a close family likeness to each other. Dr. Elam states in 'A Physician's Problem,' that on the removal of the spirit duty in Norway insanity increased 50 per cent. and congenital idiocy 150 per cent. Mr. Huth quotes from Dr. Lannurien, of Morlaix in Bretagne, where he says: "I do not hesitate to attribute the greater number of cases of idiocy in this establishment to that cause," viz. alcoholism. I certainly cannot bear that out by my experience in England. Some years since, when I expressed my conviction that acute alcoholism produced a distinct form of idiocy, it was received with some questioning. I had, however, found, from conversation with M. Morel, of Rouen, that he had noticed similar facts. Dr. Ruez has observed that idiocy was very common among the miners of Westphalia, who, living apart from their wives, only came home, and generally got drunk, on their holidays.

M. Demeaux has also recorded parallel cases. Dr. Delasiauve says that in the village of Carême, whose riches were its vineyards, the inhabitants were forced to be a little more sober in consequence of ten years' vine disease. This, he says, had a sensible effect in diminishing the cases of idiocy. Demeaux assured himself that of thirty-six epileptic patients he had under his observation for twelve years, and whose history he was able to trace, five were conceived in drunkenness. He observed two children of the same family suffering from congenital paraplegia whose conception also took place while the father was drunk.

I am not aware that any observations have been made with reference to the relation of malignant disease to idiocy, nor do I wish to attach more importance to it than it deserves. Nevertheless it is interesting to notice that 3 per cent. of the fathers and 5 per cent. of the mothers, in all 8 per cent. of the progenitors, died from cancer. Goître occurred in 2 per cent. of the mothers, but not once in a father.

I have made a very careful examination as to the relation of syphilis to idiocy, and my later inquiries have confirmed the opinion I have long taught, that syphilis is not an important factor in the production of idiocy. In not more than 2 per cent. are there signs of inherited syphilis. In making my investigations I have availed myself of the valuable observations made some years since by my friend and colleague Mr. Hutchinson, to whom the profession of medicine owes so much for his original researches. Dr. Shuttleworth confirms my opinion from investigation in another field.

I met with a history of epilepsy in 3 per cent. of the fathers and in 6 per cent. of the mothers. Phthisis exercises a very important influence among the progenitors. Several years ago I called the attention of the profession to this circumstance, and endeavoured to show that the peculiar form of idiocy to which I referred in my previous lecture as the Mongolian type was the outcome of a predominance of phthisis, and that it included about 10 per cent. of all idiots. I find that there is a marked history of this disease in 25 per cent. of the fathers or their immediate relatives, and the same thing occurs in 20 per cent. of the mothers.

In 23 per cent. of the cases there was a history of idiocy, mental feebleness, insanity, or other grave neurosis in one or several of the brothers and sisters.

I have already alluded to the influence of the emotional life of the mother on the embryo, but I have also a large mass of evidence tending to show that just as intemperance at the time of procreation may eventuate in degenerate offspring, so various kinds of mental perturbation of the father at that time may so result. I have, for example, several instances of the father begetting healthy children, except when he was the subject of recurrent mania, when idiocy resulted to the children conceived at that time. In like manner I have examples of healthy children being produced except when the merchant's business speculations have been hazardous, when the clergyman's parish has been disturbed, or the dissenting minister's church meetings have been stormy.

There are many facts which tend to indicate that the mental condition of the embryo takes its impression from the mental condition of the father at conception, and that there is a markedly varying potentiality in the sperm-cell.

It would be a very interesting question to

determine how far various trades and professions were allied with idiot offspring. I have carefully investigated the matter but have arrived at the conviction that I could not, from my cases, although very numerous, draw any very safe deductions. My patients have come from all parts of the British dominions, and include every variety of social rank, but still I am conscious that a very unfair proportion must have been drawn from this great city, that although I may have accumulated a fair number of histories from agricultural, I am sure there is a deficiency of a due proportion of cases from manufacturing districts, the great bulk having come from the southern counties of England and only a small proportion having come to me from the great manufacturing centres. I therefore feel I am unable to draw any very safe deductions with regard to the influence of employments generally in the production of, or alliance with, feeble-mindedness. Still there is a possibility of comparing the relative association of this affliction with the different professional classes, and especially with what are termed the three learned professions.

I have collected from my notes four hundred

cases with fair social antecedents, and I find that 75 per cent. are the children of merchants, country gentlemen, officers in the army and navy, gentlemen of independent means and liberal education, and members of the titled aristocracy. No less a proportion than 25 per cent. are the children of members of one or other of the three learned professions, a proportion which I take to be extremely large. On analysing still further the cases supplied by these three professions, I find that 3 per cent. are the children of lawyers while 4 per cent. are the children of members of my own profession. The remarkable circumstance, however, in the investigation is that no less than 18 per cent. are the children of members of the clerical profession. Mr. Galton has made some interesting investigations from an opposite standpoint. He takes the members of the councils of some of the prominent scientific societies of London, such as the Royal, the Linnæan, the Geological, &c, and makes the very fair inference that the 100 Members of the Councils of such Societies may be taken to be men of marked scientific attainments and of intellectual prowess. He inquires into the various professions of the men who have had such representative offshoots. He finds that the legal profession, which, according to my statistics, procreates fewest idiots, gives birth to 11 per cent. of the foremost men of eminence; that the medical profession with its 4 per cent. of idiots, gives origin to only 9 per cent. of scientific men, while the clergy, who have the maximum amount of idiocy, give birth to only 6 per cent. of men of science. In other words, while lawyers give origin to nearly three times as many scientific men as do the clergy, the clergy, on the other hand, beget six times as many feeble-minded children as do lawyers. Now, I venture to suggest that there is more than a mere accident in this. I bring it forward because, interesting in itself, it is also interesting in the support it gives to the theory that a process of natural selection has been taking place.

The life of the lawyer is such as to aggregate to that profession men of strong resolve, of mental and physical vigour, men who must be conscious that it is an avocation in which they must bring to their aid an imperturbable will and a good digestion. In the medical profession there is a larger average of moderate success. The race is not so urgent and the claims not so imperious; an aggregation of feebler elements is likely to ensue. But in the clerical profession a moderate success is still more ensured, and there is less claim among the rank and file for great mental and physical exertion. It is a profession which draws towards it many good men, but whose goodness need not be the outcome of great mental or physical power. Moreover, when once within the boundary of the Church, their usefulness and success may be in direct proportion to their retirement from intellectual turmoil, and to their assiduous cultivation of the amenities of life. It is a profession which, by its very gentleness, is likely to draw to its enclosure less the powerful will, the vigorous thought, and the ratiocinative brain, than those with bodies weak and emotions strong; men who may be classed as gently good rather than as grandly great.

The influence of marriage of consanguinity on the production of idiocy has engaged much consideration. There is a strong popular bias in favour of the theory that marriages of consanguinity are an unmixed evil, and that they are always subversive of physical and mental perfection. Mr. Huth has, however, in his classical work on the marriages of near kin, brought an amount of evidence on the other side of the question which should make us hesitate before we dogmatise on the subject.

About twenty years since I investigated the matter, and have ever since kept it prominently before me. I must confess that I approached the question with a strong bias in favour of the popular opinion. My inquiries, however, led me to see that the whole subject was worthy of reconsideration. The data on which accurate calculations can be made are unfortunately wanting, inasmuch as there is great uncertainty as to the number of people born who are the children of first cousins. I hope that at the next census this may be remedied, and that we may have reliable information on which to build more conclusive arguments. We want to know how many healthy and capable people, men and women who are doing the world's work, are the children of cousins, before we can determine what, if any, influence the marriage of cousins has in producing mental feebleness. In the absence of such data I made inquiries among the out-patients at the London

Hospital, and found ·5 per cent only were the children of cousins. It is true that my area was a limited one, and it is possible that the percentage is a low one. However, the people I did meet with who claimed to be the product of consanguineous marriages were wonderfully fine specimens of humanity. They were, as a whole, really above the average in physique and vigour. I made similar investigations among the employés in an institution, and found approximately the same result. Other inquirers, however, have made their results rather higher, and have, therefore, in like proportion *weakened* the argument against consanguineous unions. Thus, M. Boudin, using the French official returns from 1853 to 1859 inclusive, says that of every 100 mixed marriages, there were 9 consanguineous, while from another official return of marriages in France in the years 1863 to 1865, of every 100 mixed marriages 1·28 were consanguineous. M. Dalby has shown that having regard to the records obtained in the offices of the Mairie at Paris, that the results obtained both by M. Boudin and myself are probably too low, and that 1·4 per cent. is the proportion of consanguineous marriages in

Paris, a larger percentage than that derived from the official returns of France generally. Mr. George Darwin, in a paper read before the Statistical Society, endeavours to arrive at approximate results by a calculation based on the number of same name marriages, and comes to the conclusion that the ratio of consanguineous marriages in London is 1·5 per cent. and in country districts 2·75 per cent. Having regard, therefore, to results arrived at by different observers, I think that until we have more authoritative data, 1 per cent. may be taken as the percentage of marriage of first cousins. Dr. Arthur Mitchell, C.B., estimates them, at a rough guess, on the basis of his inquiries in Scotland at 1·5 per cent.

Mr. Huth marshals a great many facts to prove the position which he takes. He has no difficulty in appealing to the early history of the world to show that consanguineous marriages were the rule. Close intermarriage was practised by the great founders of the Hebrew race. Among the Ancient Egyptians and Persians he indicates that incestuous marriages were common in the kings and people of high rank without apparently any evil result, and he shows by numberless appeals to Athenian and Spartan history how frequent, and yet how harmless, was marriage of near-of-kin. The whole question has been discussed with an amount of partisanship, which is very remarkable. One disputant goes so far as to attribute hydatids in the liver to consanguineous unions, others again charge to marriages of near kin " organic degeneration fatal to the propagation of the species."

Dr. Shuttleworth has recently published a paper on the subject, in which he discusses the question with marked moderation. His statistics, gathered in the North of England, are slightly different from mine, gathered in the South, and are on the surface less significant of the danger of the unions we are discussing than were mine. Although I have no doubt of the care with which Dr. Shuttleworth's cases were taken, there is always a danger of the friends not appreciating the question, or of desiring to conceal the relationship, and so making the percentage of births from the union of cousins too low. They are not so likely to exaggerate the percentage by the assertion of a relationship which does not exist. In a careful examination of 852 cases of known parentage I found that 60 were children of consanguineous marriages, or at the rate of 7 per cent., while among these 46 or 5·4, per cent., were first cousins. Dr. Shuttleworth, in analysing 900 cases, found that 5·1 per cent. were consanguineous marriages, and of these 2·9 per cent. first cousin marriages. While Dr. Shuttleworth finds that 5 is the average number of children born to relatives who have intermarried, I find that the average number of children born under like circumstances is 6·9. It will be observed that the latter figures are not far removed from the average of my 2000 cases, which is 7, so that there is not much to be said as to consanguineous marriages being less prolific than others. I am conscious, moreover, in considering my statistics and those of Dr. Shuttleworth, that I am comparing things which are not the same; his cases do not include epileptic children, whereas mine do. This may account in some measure for the disparity. Since I wrote on the subject twenty years ago I have continued making observations, and have no reason to materially alter the percentages at which I then arrived. I have recently gone over the notes of 400 fresh cases; they have been taken with great care, and I am certain that no error has crept in. Of the 400, 26 were children of consanguineous unions, or $6\frac{1}{2}$ per cent., a difference so small as rather to confirm the value of my statistics on the larger number. Nineteen of these were the children of first cousins, or 4·75 per cent.; 6 were children of second cousins, and 1 of third. When I came to analyse my cases further I was struck with the obvious causes of their feeble-mindedness, other than the marriage of near kin, which the notes of my cases brought to light. I took out of my portfolio 20 unselected cases, and on examining the life-history of their progenitors, I found that in 1 only was the consanguinity of the parents the only discoverable factor. I am convinced that frequently the absence of investigation into the other possible factors has led to such contradictory opinions on this subject. Take an illustration from my notes culled by chance from my portfolio.

J. T. W—, born in the parish of St. Luke's, 1866. His father is a lever escapement maker, his mother worked as a tailoress before her marriage. Father always subject to headache and to dizziness, frequently to fainting. Mother dreadfully nervous; her uncle died insane; had a cousin imbecile; the grandmother also was extremely nervous.

He is the first-born child and had five brothers; two have died, one from a fit during whooping-cough, and the other from bronchitis; one of those living is paralysed; another, three years and five months old, cannot talk. His father fell down in a fainting fit (epilepsy?) which frightened his mother very much when five months advanced in pregnancy and brought on uterine hæmorrhage. We read further that the father and mother were first cousins, but it is absurd to suppose that this was the most important factor in the production of the child's idiocy. No one could contemplate the union of two such persons, whether related or not, without predicting disastrous results to their progeny. Although looked at superficially my statistics are rather less favorable to the marriage of first cousins than are those of many other observers, I am strongly of opinion that, having regard to the remarkable antecedent neurotic history of the first cousins who have married and procreated feeble-minded children, the evil apparently resulting is that where there is hereditary predisposition the intermarriage of relations determines the concurrence of two morbid factors, and this may account for the undoubted greater frequency of feeble-minded children among the progeny of cousins than among those of mixed marriages. My views are quite in harmony with those of Dr. Charles Withington, who regards morbid inheritance rather than specific degenerative tendencies as accounting for all infirmities met with in the offspring of cousins.

It is interesting to note that Dr. Kerlin, of Pennsylvania, a remarkably accurate observer, arrives at precisely the same conclusion as I have, that 7 per cent. of feeble-minded people are the children of consanguineous marriages.

Dr. Voisin made a careful examination of 1077 of his patients at Bicêtre and Salpêtrière, and in no instance could healthy consanguinity be regarded as the cause of idiocy, epilepsy, or insanity.

I have thus endeavoured to show that while the marriage of cousins insures a degenerate offspring where there is something morbid in the family history—where phthisis, scrofula, and especially the neuroses exist, I am by no means sure that by a judicious selection of cousins the race might not be improved. Dr. Clouston thinks there seems to be a special tendency for members of neurotic families to intermarry, and that an affective affinity amongst such tends to love and marriage. I must say that my experience, on the contrary, would rather lead me to agree with Mr. Grant Allen that "what we each fall in love with individually, is our moral, mental, and physical complement." The intermarriage of cousins arises in all probability from their seeing and knowing more of one another, without committing themselves to an engagement, than can be possible in ordinary life. Other things being equal, I cannot but believe that the physiological law is more usually followed, seeking our unlike and our opposite. However that may be, there is no strong argument, in my opinion, to be based on an inquiry into the etiology of idiocy in favour of the doctrine that consanguinity *per se* is an important factor in the production of the evil, and that this doctrine is held is shown by the writings of Devay, of Lyons, who asserted "that in pure consanguinity, isolated from all circumstances of hereditary disease, resides, *ipso facto*, a principle of organic vitiation." Commencing the investigation twenty years ago, and continuing it up to the present time, I am able to agree with Dr. Shuttleworth, that if a close scrutiny does not reveal any hereditary weakness, neurotic or otherwise, that the facts and figures alone will not in all instances justify us in "forbidding the banns."

Illegitimacy has been regarded as a cause of idiocy. Dr. Arthur Mitchell, from statistics taken in Scotland, where illegitimacy appears to be frequent, came to the conclusion that it is a very common cause. He supports the probability of this by reference to the superior viability of legitimate as compared with illegitimate children. Thus at Berlin every twenty-fifth child of the legitimate and every twelfth child of the illegitimate were stillborn, and after birth the mortality of the legitimate before the age of five years is to that of the illegitimate as 6 to 3.

I cannot but think that these statistics are open to another explanation. My own investigations do not throw much light on the subject, because my 2000 cases are mainly from children born in wedlock, the illegitimate cases finding their way into the workhouses. Among the few that have come under my notice where there was reason to suspect their legitimacy, there has been enough in the anxieties of the mother's position to account for the disaster. With the prospect of giving birth to a child with a compromised position one cannot wonder that the agony of mind incident to it, should arrest the development of the embryo and give rise either to congenital or developmental idiocy. I am quite prepared, therefore, to expect that in a different class than that from which my statistics are drawn illegitimacy may be a potent *emotional* factor.

Attempts to produce abortion have been also regarded as a cause, and it is possible that this may be one among others to add to the numbers of feeble-minded children the outcome of illegitimacy. I am, however, not able from my personal experience to confirm or negative the statement.

Idiocy is occasionally induced by deprivation of the senses. The case of Laura Bridgman (although not an idiot) has become known wherever the English language is spoken, as a triumph of the perseverance of the late Dr. Howe over difficulties which seemed insurmountable. I have had one such example under my care. The subject of the deprivation was a boy who could neither see, hear, nor speak, and this deprivation was from birth. He had a very acute sense of touch and that of smell was equally good. He knew by their odour all those who were brought into daily relation with him, and caressed lovingly those who ministered to his wants in the way of food and warmth. Attempts were made to teach him to associate actions with things, especially articles of food. I tried to teach him a sign for sugar (of which he was very fond) by the movement of the hand in a vertical direction, but without success, although it was repeated again and again with most persevering efforts. It was, unfortunately, a case in which there was a damaged cerebrum, and he became epileptic. It was most remarkable, however, how at once he smelled out his friends and manifested by a smile his consciousness of their proximity. That smile was always a reproof to us, who had full possession of our senses, for our occasional petulence at things of minor import, while this deprived boy never whined but appeared delighted at the most insignificant creature comforts.

There is a very important class of cases which owes its origin to malaria or other endemic causes, and which is called Cretinism. A great deal of attention has been given to this disease, and I have had the opportunity of studying it myself in the Italian Valley of Aosta. Here I found it in greater profusion than in any of the valleys of the Bavarian or Swiss Alps. The fact that cretinism is not confined to the valleys of mountainous regions but is found also along the course of the great rivers, suggests the probability of its having a malarial origin. Every variety of theory has been resorted to, from the presence of iron in the water to the presence of magnesia. Cretinism is not unknown in England, and has been found in Derbyshire and some parts of Yorkshire, I have seen several cases coming from one part of Somersetshire, not to be distinguished in their general features from those met with in the Swiss and Italian valleys. Virchow and Zillner both trace a connexion between marsh fever and acute affections of the thyroid gland. Certain it is that, while the goîtrous people are not necessarily cretins, the race tends by a process of gradual deterioration to cretinism. A large number of cretins met with in the Valley of Aosta were not goîtrous in the least degree, but their grandparents, who were not cretins, had enormous thyroid glands and the peculiar tawny look which is characteristic of cretinism as well as of palludal poisoning. Cretinism is, however, met with in England sporadically. My colleague, Mr. T. B. Curling, was the first to call the attention of the profession to these cases, in the year 1850. Without having been aware of his paper I brought a case before the Pathological Society in 1869, having had cases under my observation from the year 1860. I have now had altogether twelve sporadic cretins under my care, and in the majority there was reason to believe that they were procreated during the intemperance of the father, some of the later ones could not have been procreated under any other condition. They all had a very great resemblance to each other, most of them had their growth arrested at the period of first dentition, in three of the number, however, growth was not arrested until the period of second dentition. They all had two characteristics; there was no evidence of the presence of a thyroid gland, and they all had puffy swellings, which Mr. Curling showed to be fatty, in the supraclavicular spaces. In a case I have recently had under my care, and who died a few months since from tubercular meningitis, the supraclavicular swellings entirely disappeared before death. Apparently it was a reserve stock of fatty material, which vanished with the general emaciation. The characteristics of these children are their extreme placidity, they are unruffled in temper, seldom cry, never shed tears. They are imitative and have a strong sense of humour. Their speech is usually deferred, and when acquired is monosyllabic. They are orderly and precise, disturbed by anything out of the usual routine. Their skin has a wrinkled appearance, as if too large for their diminutive bodies. Their faces have an earthy colour. The hair is commonly sparse, and they suffer from pityriasis of the scalp. They have usually a large development of areolar tissue, and two of my cases were characterised by polysarcia, one weighing 210 lbs.

Three of my twelve cases were males, nine

were females. They all had brachycephalic crania, flattened noses, and the distances of the inner canthi exaggerated. Their tongues were large for their mouths, and their lips were thick. There was in the majority a tendency to suck their tongues. In three only was there much intellectual response to teaching. They were all, however, with one exception, readily taught to be clean in their habits, making signs to indicate their natural wants. Menstruation had not appeared even in those who had reached the years of womanhood, and the external organs of generation were infantile in appearance, and apparently there was complete absence of sexual instinct.

In the year 1857, M. Baillarger presented a case of sporadic cretinism before the Société Medico-Psychologique of Paris, and described it as a very remarkable one. It is a girl, he said, born at Melun, of healthy and well-formed parents. The first dentition was completed at three years of age, and it was then that general development was arrested. The girl is now about twenty-seven, and she has the intelligence and tastes of a child of four or five; she plays with a doll, and has no sentiments of modesty.

After describing the characteristics of the case, which resemble very closely those which I have detailed as being common to mine, he goes on to say that the body is fat, the limbs thick and short and sufficiently regular; the second dentition only commenced at eighteen, and has not yet terminated. The pubis is smooth, the mammary glands rudimentary; menstruation has not been established, and there has never been any sexual sensation. M. Baillarger throws out the suggestion that the condition of this case, and of another that he had seen in Paris with M. Rayer, arose from inactivity of the generative organs.

The relation between goître and cretinism is of extreme interest. The late Dr. Hilton Fagge in 1871 regarded goître and cretinism to be antagonistic effects of the same cause. He suggested that when the cause acts with little intensity the sole effect is goître, but if it acts with great intensity or upon successive generations it at length produces cretinism as well as goître. The not infrequent absence of goître in cretins, when not dependent upon congenital deficiency of the thyroid body, must, he thought, be attributable to some local morbid change in it, by which it is prevented from undergoing enlargement under the operation of the morbific agent. He suggested that when goître has existed in a family for two or three generations, the structure of the thyroid body may undergo deterioration in members of the succeeding generation. When we have regard to the remarkable cases of cretinoid changes in adult women described so well by Sir William Gull, and the many examples which have been since accumulated by many observers, and especially by Dr. Ord and Sir Dyce Duckworth, we cannot fail to see the close relation between cretinism and degenerative changes in the thyroid. This is further strengthened by the fact made known to us by Professor Kocher, of Berne, that after the removal of the thyroid for goître, a condition gradually supervenes which much resembles adult cretinism, while Professor Horsley, operating on monkeys by removal of their thyroids, has produced symptoms resembling myxœdema which, by virtue of the increase of mucin in the tissues, is the name which has been proposed to be given to the cretinoid condition described by Sir William Gull. It is very noticeable that many of the physical as well as mental and moral characteristics of myxœdema resemble those of sporadic cretinism, and, like it, occur mostly in women. The only exception I have seen was a cabdriver brought by Dr. Fenn, of Richmond, before a meeting of the Thames Valley branch of the British Medical Association. I cannot but feel that the inquiries which are being made with regard to myxœdema will eventually throw light on the etiology of endemic and sporadic cretinism.

There is one subject of great interest at the present time which is made the topic of addresses from presidential chairs as well as of numerous articles in periodical literature. I mean the higher education of women. The doctrine which has been promulgated of late is, that the higher culture of the faculties of women will make them less capable of becoming "mothers of men." There has been hitherto no objection to their being taught everything relating to art, music, or their emotional life, but directly there are attempts made to cultivate their judgment, to teach them how to reason, to inculcate habits of self-control, we are met by clamours which, in my opinion, are not based on experience, and, so far as the etiology of feeble-mindedness is concerned, are likely to be prejudicial. If there is one thing more certain than another about the production of idiocy it is the danger which arises from the culture of only one side of a woman's nature; so long as only the emotional side of their nature is cultivated and they are responsive to the least unexpected sound, unreasoning as to the world of nature about them, and thrown into emotional paroxysms by the sights and trials which will be sure to cross their path, they will, from my point of view, be liable to become the mothers of idiots. Without advocating over-pressure, which is as bad for the neurotic boy as for the neurotic girl, and which is to be avoided during the developmental life of the one as well as during the developmental life of the other, there can be no reason why the faculties which they possess should not be cultivated so as to make them not only fit to be " mothers of men " but also companions and helpers of men. At all events, let the trial be made without prejudice, and let us welcome the advent of a time when women shall not be the mere frivolous toys of the hour but have and enjoy the privileges and rights of which it is absurd to deprive them.

My statistics show that we must look mainly to the health and mental life of the parents. They point to the importance of training our sons to be temperate and our daughters to be self-possessed. They indicate that we should seek alliances for our daughters with men from a healthy stock, that our sons should avoid women whose emotions are developed at the sacrifice of their judgment and self-control. They show that idiocy is often the natural outcome of a gradual process in which the strain becomes more and more degenerate, requiring only an insignificant factor to produce the direst results.

LECTURE III.

*Infantile Mania.—Melancholia and Delusions.—Moral Insanity.
—" Idiots Savants."—Variations in the Mental Condition.
—Epilepsy and Catalepsy.—Physical Deformities.—Associated Diseases.—Rate of Growth.—Diagnosis of Idiocy.—
" Backward Children."—Deferred or Absent Speech.—
Morbid Anatomy.—Treatment of Feeble-mindedness.*

INFANTILE mania is not of frequent occurrence and has not been the subject of much comment. Nevertheless very well-marked examples have come under my notice in quite young children; cases where the various phases of insanity in the adult have been well represented; acute maniacal attacks, in which the patient tears and destroys everything within reach, or creeps under tables and sofas to hide, screaming with undisguised rage and biting and scratching anyone who approaches. This attack subsides and the boy behaves as nicely and intelligently as possible, but in a few days has a recurrence with as great violence as before. Some few years since a little boy of this class was sent to me. He was by no means deficient in mental acuteness, in many respects was precocious; he was an only child, and having lived a good deal with adult people he talked rather sagely, but he was liable to attacks of acute mania of a very marked kind. There were no bounds to his petulance and violence. He would attack his father in the street and behave in all respects in an insane manner, regardless of any injury he might inflict, even on those for whom he ordinarily entertained affection. In the intervals of the paroxysms he manifested traits which made him much liked by those about him.

Occasionally I have met with cases having well-marked delusions of suspicion. The ordinary trust and unsuspiciousness of childhood has been replaced by painful mistrust. In one case the child imagined that he was watched and that someone was listening at the key-hole. Another had delusions that things were mixed with his food and had evident fear of being poisoned. I have seen some cases of melancholia associated with manifest delusions, one boy believing that he resembled an animal and frequently looking into the mirror to confirm or dissipate the conviction; another believed that she would break if you touched her, and the fear of falling to pieces like a fragile piece of glass was a real terror to her. I had some years since under my observation a girl who, when eight years of age, put her baby brother on the fire so that he was dreadfully burnt. The girl herself was ill-favoured in appearance and she had been accustomed to hear the beauty of her brother injudiciously praised. In a maniacal attack she attempted to get rid of the subject of so much laudation. About three years subsequently she became epileptic and again later on the subject of epileptic dementia. It is highly probable that the maniacal paroxysm which manifested itself in homicidal mania was really masked epilepsy.

As puberty approaches attacks of mental aberration assume a special character; there is frequently unnatural introspection and a critical hyper-conscientiousness becomes prominent. I have recently had five cases under my care, three boys and two girls. They have all had characters much in common, they have all been very good and studious children, but between eleven and thirteen years of age have become moody, have had conscientious scruples as to their motives, have been anxious not only as to whether they have told the truth, but whether when having told it, they have done so in such a way as to convey to others the precise idea in their minds. They have had morbid views as to the standard of right and wrong; sometimes they have detailed things in a non-sequential way. One boy was troubled when he saw a dirty beggar-man or boy lest he should contaminate his mother by thinking of her immediately afterwards. I saw him greatly perturbed one day from having seen an errand-boy come to the school-house, and his thoughts flitting to his mother he was rendered inexpressibly miserable lest he had lowered, injured, and contaminated her by unwittingly thinking at the same time of her and the dirty boy. I have sometimes known an avoidance of anything positive in assertion lest the exact truth should not be spoken, so that all the replies are, "Perhaps it was," "It may have been," "I may have done so and so," about things in which no principle was involved, but from a morbid fear of not saying what was true. These cases cause great anxiety at the time and occasionally lead to a permanent breakdown. Many, however, by careful management may be tided over the climacteric period of puberty and then all may go well. It is important, however, to be on guard against any concealed suicidal impulse, and to note its slightest indication, as the tendency in such cases is to melancholia and in some instances temptation to self-inflicted injury. Care should also be taken to be quite sure that there is no sexual deviation, and if there be, to treat it, not as moral wrong, which would inevitably lead to further mental disquietude and peril, but as a physical evil which, for the good of the body, it is important should be corrected. These deviations are readily recognised by the aggregation of a group of symptoms which rarely leads one astray. They are, supra-orbital headache, dilated pupils, a brown-umber areola surrounding the eyes, an averted look and a statuesque bearing. This last symptom alone is often very conclusive and may be regarded as certain if associated with the preceding; occasionally the statuesqueness is so marked as to resemble a minor cataleptic state.

Moral insanity is met with in childhood and youth. It has fallen to my lot to have had a great many illustrations brought under my notice—cases of purposeless theft, purposeless lying, and purposeless mischief. They are difficult cases to treat, and make great demands on one's resources. The subjects of this condition are sometimes intellectually bright, and have an amount of address which makes them extremely troublesome to their friends and those who have to guide them. I was consulted some years since about a boy who displayed such destructive energies on toys and every household appliance that he could get into his possession, that his friends thought it indicated a latent mechanical talent, and as he had also manifested mathematical ability he was apprenticed to a firm of engineers. Here his pleasure in creating astonishment led him to introduce sand into the mechanism of the machinery he had to overlook, apparently getting amusement out of the consternation and inquiry which his evil deeds induced. He managed for some time to conceal his delinquency by clever lies; but at length the mischief was fastened on him from his having allowed a traversing machine to go beyond its support in order that he might see the mischief that would ensue. He had good musical talent, and acquiring some skill as an organ player, he would play occasionally in church, and suddenly stop to enjoy the discomfiture his irregularity produced. Eventually he became a thief and was several times in danger of being brought under the criminal law. All his delinquencies were conceived and carried out with great skill; there was no intellectual lesion, but his moral and affective faculties were thoroughly dormant. He saw no wrong in what he did and he entertained no affection for his parents, who were in a state of perpetual agony. Had he been a member of a lower stratum of society he would have become a jail-bird. Great pains were taken to prevent his getting into the hands of the police, and, the period of puberty passed, he has reached manhood with improved moral sense, and is now getting his living by his musical talent in a respectable and honorable way.

More frequently moral insanity is associated in children and youths with some amount of mental backwardness. The backwardness may be very slight, but yet sufficient to prevent their taking appropriate place in form or in the playground. The manifestations of moral insanity in such cases are multiform. I have seen a boy who had brought from school sixteen watches without being discovered by the sufferers or the principal of the school, and this so cleverly done as for a long time to elude detection. Another was dismissed from school because he persisted in getting on the roof and putting pillows and other articles of bedding down the chimneys of neighbouring houses in the terrace, or in filling the pillar boxes with stones. Another would beg sufficient money during the morning in the streets to enable him to travel backward and forward by the Underground Railway the whole of the remainder of the day. A still more dangerous form is a tendency sometimes met with of setting fire to articles of furniture, often where it would be perilous to themselves as well as others. Many forms of low cunning are developed in backward boys by associating them with others with more wit, who are also bullies, the feebler one calling to his aid lying, theft, and deceit, to compensate for his lessened intellectual vigour. Again and again I have seen the moral sense developed in boys of this class when they have been removed from the bullying to which they had been subjected and submitted to appropriate training. In all the cases I have met with of moral insanity there has been marked antecedent neurotic history.

This is a convenient place to treat of an interesting class of cases for which the term "idiots savants" has been given, and of which a considerable number have come under my observation. This name has been applied to children who, while feeble-minded, exhibit special faculties which are capable of being cultivated to a very great extent. One youth was under my care who could build exquisite model ships from drawings, and carve with a great deal of skill, who yet could not understand a sentence —who had to have it dissected for him, and who, when writing to his mother copied *verbatim* a letter from 'The Life of Captain Hedley Vicars,' by Miss Marsh, although it had not the slightest appropriateness in word or sentiment. Another has been under my care who can draw in crayons with marvellous skill and feeling, in whom nevertheless there was a comparative blank in all the higher faculties of mind.

Extraordinary memory is often met with associated with very great defect of reasoning power. A boy came under my observation who, having once read a book, could ever more remember it. He would recite all the answers in 'Magnall's Questions' without an error, giving in detail the numbers in the astronomical division with the greatest accuracy. I discovered, however, that it was simply a process of verbal adhesion. I once gave him Gibbon's 'Rise and Fall of the Roman Empire' to read. This he did, and on reading the third page he skipped a line, found out his mistake and retraced his steps; ever after, when reciting from memory the stately periods of Gibbon, he would, on coming to the third page, skip the line and go back and correct the error with as much regularity as if it had been part of the regular text. Later on his memory for recent reading became less tenacious, but his recollection of his earlier readings never failed him. Another boy can tell the tune, words, and number of nearly every hymn in 'Hymns Ancient and Modern.' Often the memory takes the form of remembering dates and past events. Several children under my observation have had this faculty in an extraordinary degree. One boy never fails to be able to tell the name and address of every confectioner's shop that he has visited in London—and they have been numerous—and can as readily tell the date of every visit. Another can tell the time of arrival of all the children at an institution, and could supply accurate records in relation to it if needed. Another knows the home address of every resident who comes under his observation, and they are by no means few. The faculty of number is usually slightly developed with feeble-minded children while memory is fairly well developed, and yet I have had under my observation cases where the power of mental arithmetic existed to an astonishing extent. One boy, about twelve years of age, could multiply any three figures by three figures with perfect accuracy, and as quickly as I could write the six figures on paper, and yet, so low mentally was he, that although having been for two and a half years in almost the daily habit of seeing me and talking to me, could not tell my name. Another boy who has recently been under my observation can multiply two figures by two figures, while another can multiply rapidly two figures by two, and a short time since could multiply three figures by three figures, but since an epileptiform attack has lost this faculty to some extent. None of them can explain how they do it, I mean, by what mental process. When by rare chance they have made a mistake, and some hesitation has arisen, it has appeared to me, the plan has been, to clear off the multiplication of the higher figures first. Improvisation is an occasional faculty. I had a boy under my care who could take up a book, pretending to read, an art he had not acquired, and improvise stories of all kinds with a great deal of skill, and in any variety, to suit the supposed tastes of his auditors.

Memory of tune is a very common faculty among the feeble-minded; they readily acquire simple airs, and rarely forget them. I have had one boy under my observation who, if he went to an opera, would carry away a recollection of all the airs, and would hum or sing them correctly. In none of the cases of "idiot savant" have I been able to trace any history of a like faculty in the parents or in the brothers and sisters, nor have I had any opportunity of making an autopsy, except in one instance. This was in the case of a boy who had a very unusual faculty, of which I have never since met another example, viz. the perfect appreciation of past or passing time. He was seventeen years of age, and although not understanding, so far as I could gather, the use of a clock-face, could tell the time to a minute at any part of the day, and in any situation. I tried him on numberless occasions, and he always answered with an amount of precision truly remarkable. Gradually his response became less ready, and he would not or could not reply unless he was a little excited. He had to be shaken like an old watch, and then the time would be truly given. Gradually his health became enfeebled and the faculty departed. At an autopsy I found that there was no difference in his cerebrum from an ordinary brain, except that he had two well-marked and distinct soft commissures. My explanation of the phenomenon was that as every movement in the house was absolutely punctual he had data from which he could estimate the time by accurate appreciation of its flux. All these cases of "idiots savants" were males; I have never met with a female.

It happens to the congenitally feeble-minded as to the strong-minded to have deviations from their normal standard. There is therefore every form of mental aberration to be met with among them. They become the subjects of acute and chronic mania, of acute and chronic melancholia, and of dementia. It is curious to witness the change which may take place in the mental and moral condition of one deprived to a great extent of intellectual power. Feeble-minded children are not naturally suicidal; they are liable to meet with accidents from their not having any sense of fear, or from not being able to work out the logical sequence of any act, but, under the influence of a melancholic state, they do sometimes become suicidal. Occasionally, under the influence of acute mania, the feeble intellect of the youth becomes fanned into a brighter flame, and he may say things which are quite in advance of his ordinary powers, becoming for the time quick in repartee or pertly rude. The taciturn may become loquacious, the timid and respectful proud and defiant, and the amiable and tractable abusive and destructive. Occasionally, too, a remarkable change takes place in those who are temporarily the subject of the delirium of fever. Three remarkable instances have occurred to me of boys who had never been heard to speak, making use of well-formed sentences during the high febrile state of acute pneumonia in two instances, and of scarlatina in another. In the case of one, who was the subject of pneumonia, the other boys who were in the Infirmary at the time were frightened by the febrile ejaculation of their usually speechless companion.

There are two ailments from which, according to my experience, the congenitally feeble-minded are remarkably free, viz. chorea and hysteria. I cannot call to mind, among the large number of cases that have come under my notice, a single case of acute chorea. I have met with cases of chronic and persistent inco-ordinated movements, but not with the acute cases so common in a general hospital or in a hospital for children. I have assumed that it is partly owing to the lessened emotional life of my patients. The same reason may account for the rare occurrence of hysteria. This defective emotional element in the feeble-minded spares them much grief. Although very affectionate, they will hear of the loss of beloved relations or friends without emotional disturbance and with a remarkable philosophy. They live very much in the present, and are not perturbed by the troubles of the past or the unexperienced future.

Epilepsy is a very common complication of feeble-mindedness. Of the whole number that have come under my observation, 24 per cent. have been at some period of their lives epileptic. This appears to be a very large average and indicates to what a great extent the treatment of idiocy is the treatment of epilepsy. Dr. Kerlin, of Pennsylvania, states that "from an examination of the history of 300 imbecile children between the ages of five and sixteen, I find that 66, or 22 per cent., are now epileptics." The percentage is so near my own as to confirm very materially my observations. My cases, however, are not within equally narrow limits as to age, but range from two years to forty. Dr. Kerlin further confirms my observations as to the important neurotic antecedents of feeble-minded children, when he states that 52 per cent. have in their antecedents the history of the epileptoid family of diseases. A large number fall under the developmental class and are often associated with a history of eclampsia at first dentition. I have frequently observed attacks come on during second dentition, followed by an interval of freedom until the evolution of puberty. Epilepsy often appears for the first time at puberty and subsequently ceases. Occasionally the status epilepticus supervenes with the worst possible results.

Catalepsy is met with among the feeble-minded, but always in my experience associated with impure habits.

The physical deviations of the feeble-minded are very important. I have already referred to the lessened common sensation and defective co-ordination to which they are prone, to their diminished sense of taste and smell, and to their sight. Hearing is often obtuse, and is, as I have said, frequently a cause of deferred speech. They are very prone to eczematous eruptions in the flexures of the joints and behind the ears. The skin gives evidence of degeneration in its tendency to unnatural unions; just as the petals of a corollifloral exogen indicate a lower grade than the distinct petals of a thalamifloral so do webbing of the fingers and toes and adhesions of the lobules of the ear suggest marked inferiority. Dr. Laycock many years ago called attention to the prevalence of ear abnormalities in people of a degenerate type, and my own observations coincide with his. Lobules absent, lobules adherent, helices defective, and the entire pinnæ misshapen or shrunken, are very common among the congenital feeble-minded. The implantation of the ear is often too far back, giving an exaggerated facial development. I have had under my observation very remarkable examples of webbing, both of toes and fingers, in all cases associated with adherent lobules of the ears. The development of the hair offers some anomalies; some are hirsute over their entire bodies, and 11 per cent. have the eyebrows continuous over the nose. I have before referred to the deformations of the mouth and the importance I attach to these in diagnosis. The tongue as a muscular organ is very ill co-ordinated, and this is one factor in the absence or defect of speech which is so characteristic of the feeble-minded. In a number of cases, taken without selection, of an age when speech would be expected, 36 per cent. may be regarded as being entirely dumb, and 30 per cent. with speech indistinct, while not more than 28 per cent. speak fluently; the remaining

6 per cent. speak a little and distinctly but with a small vocabulary. With such retarded development it is not astonishing to find that puberty is postponed on an average two years.

Mastication is often defective, partly from carious teeth, and partly from a want of persistent voluntary effort. Deglutition is often hurried, and ill-masticated food is bolted. Rumination occasionally occurs. Three well-marked examples have come under my notice; in one of the cases I found the œsophagus distinctly pouched. They all eructated their food and then placidly remasticated the mass. Excepting when asleep, these were the quietest times of their lives, being ordinarily restless and impatient. The whole process of feeding very closely resembled that of the ruminants.

There is a great tendency to swallow unusual things, such as pebbles and neckties, which generally prove quite inert. Occasionally, however, the swallowed morsels are not so innocuous, and there are now two or three deaths on record from intestinal obstruction caused by the slow accumulation of hair either bitten from their own head or extracted from mattresses or from swallowing a fibre at a time, picked out of cocoanut matting. As might be supposed from the defective innervation which characterises feeble-minded children they are neither fleet nor persistent in endurance. They are deficient in muscular power as they are also deficient in mental tension. The organs of reproduction are ill developed; among females I have found a great prevalence of small ovaries, and in the males 8 per cent. of those who have reached the age of fourteen have either undeveloped or undescended testes. In recording this estimate it is worthy of remark that both accidental, developmental, and congenital feeble-minded youths are included, and I have no doubt that if the investigation had been confined to congenital cases the percentage of defective generative organs would have been much greater.

I have omitted to speak of one very marked characteristic of the nervous system, viz. defective reflex functions. The feeble-minded are very prone to constipation, and it is extremely difficult to produce emesis; they resist any ordinary dose of an emetic nature. On the occasion of several children who had returned from a day's holiday complaining of similar pains in their stomachs, which gave rise to the suspicion that some article of food had been unwholesome, attempts were made to induce vomiting by the administration of twenty grains of sulphate of zinc to each, but in not a single case was it successful, although the fauces were also irritated by a feather. The same thing applies to the absence of cough and expectoration when they are the subjects of phthisis. It is not uncommon for a feeble-minded patient to pass through all the stages of this disease without the slightest cough. Their vaso-motor system, on the other hand, is very sensitive ; they are prone to gastric intestinal trouble from sudden change of weather, from bolting their food, from taking too much food at a meal, and from too great predominance of meat as an article of diet, or from the presence of electrical disturbance. Occasionally, but not frequently, feeble-mindedness is associated with disseminated sclerosis, with its characteristic gait and scanning speech ; more frequently, however, with pseudo-hypertrophic paralysis, two well-marked cases of which I have published in the 'Pathological Transactions,' and several others have been under my observation. In fact, I have seen but few examples of that disease which have not been also characterised by some amount of intellectual lesion. Diseases of the kidneys and liver are extremely rare, on account of the discreet and temperate habits which such patients are accustomed to lead under medical guidance. Rheumatism is very exceptional, probably from the non-exposure to bad weather which the nature of their lives induces. Putting aside the diseases of childhood, diseases of the brain and of the lungs are the chief causes of death. Having regard to the frequency of epilepsy as a complication, it is not surprising that it should be a cause of considerable mortality among the feeble-minded. I find, from the returns of Dr. Fletcher Beach, that about $2\frac{1}{2}$ per cent. of the average daily number of inmates of the schools at Darenth die from epilepsy, or more than the mortality of London from all causes whatever.

The prevalence of phthisis as a cause of death among the feeble-minded varies very much with the nature of the soil on which they reside. Through the admirable researches of Dr. G. Buchanan we now know how much associated a damp clay soil is with the existence of phthisis.

He has taught us that measures which have been taken in some towns and cities for their drainage in consequence of the prevalence of zymotic disease, have resulted in diminishing the mortality from pulmonary consumption in a remarkable degree.

My own experience lends support, if support were needed, to Dr. Buchanan's view. In the year 1867 I wrote a paper in the 'Lancet' "On the Relation of Idiocy to Tuberculosis," in which I showed how prevalent phthisis was among idiots, amounting to 39·8 per cent. of the general mortality. My experience since that time has suggested that I ought rather to have headed my paper, "On the Relation of Tuberculosis to a Clay Soil." My observations were made on 1000 feet of Wealden Clay, and I did not know at that time what a relationship existed between the two. My more recent experience on a gravel soil shows the deaths from phthisis to be only 12 per cent. of the general mortality. I concluded my paper with this paragraph: "It is no less clear to me that idiocy of a non-tubercular origin leads to tuberculosis. Whether this arises through the influence of the pneumogastric nerve, mal-assimilation of food, or defective innervation, it cannot but be regarded that the connection between these maladies is by no means accidental, and that a due appreciation of this relation is necessary to those who would treat effectively congenital mental lesions." I feel it my duty to add to this that the question of soil is an important matter which I then overlooked. When we have regard to the number of days in which outdoor exercise is impossible on a clay soil in a climate like that of England, the difficulty of draining it effectively, and the damp exhalations which the clay gives out in warm, and the mist which is condensed in cold weather, we can appreciate the effect it is likely to have on children and youths whose ordinary mortality is greater than that of those with normal nervous power and nutritive energy.

Nothing is more remarkable than the readiness with which feeble-minded children succumb to acute disease of any form, or the way in which they are injuriously affected by climatic changes. The incidence of illness should be narrowly looked for and promptly treated; the thermometer is of great value in indicating the need of early precautionary measures. Before the introduction of the clinical thermometer the principal indication of deviation from health was loss of appetite. I have known a boy in whose case the first suggestion of illness consisted of a face suffused with tears, because, as he said, the boy who had sat next him at tea had eaten three slices of bread and butter and he could not eat any. This was the prelude to one of the most serious ailments to which the feeble-minded are subject, namely, broncho-pneumonia.

My own observations as regards the height and weight of idiots are very much in harmony with those of Dr. Shuttleworth, and Dr. Tarbell of America. I find that feeble-minded children are shorter and lighter than the normal standard, and agree with Mr. Charles Roberts, "that the relative rate of growth of the two sexes of idiot children follows the same rule as that of normal children, and is subject to the same variations at the age of puberty." "It was found by Dr. Bowditch," so writes Dr. Tarbell, "in his investigation of normal children, that until the age of eleven or twelve years boys are both taller and heavier than girls of the same age. At this period of life girls begin to grow very rapidly, and for the next two or three years surpass boys of the same age both in height and weight. Boys then acquire and retain a size superior to that of girls, who have now nearly completed their full growth."

The diagnosis of idiocy is of importance, both in order that the child may early be put under proper training and for medico-legal purposes. The profound cases are not difficult to diagnose, especially if associated with microcephalism or with marked asymmetry of cranium. The congenital class is that which has to be considered in early life. There is a marked want of muscular power, as indicated by the inability to support the head and to use the hands for prehension. The eyes look out as if on an objectless world, and the attention is not arrested by the usual expedients to excite recognition in infants. To the most loving endearments there is no responsive smile, and the infantile cooing is replaced by a wailing cry. The instinctive process of feeding is often acquired with difficulty and indicates, what I have long observed, that there is no predominance of instinct in idiocy. On the contrary, so far as instinct itself is concerned, the young animal is on a higher platform than an idiot baby. The latter would not search out the source of the maternal supply nor make successful efforts to regain the nipple if once out of the mouth. Later on there is a marked indisposition to make muscular effort, there is no responsive leap when the feet are allowed to touch the ground, and when taken in the hands the scapular muscles offer no resistance, and the arms helplessly extend themselves over the head. There is no disposition to crawl but rather to lie on the back in an irresolute way. Still later the power of standing is deferred, and walking is an accomplishment which may never be attained.

I have already referred to the physical deviations in congenital idiots, such as the deformed cranium, the vaulted palate, and ill-developed ears, and these come to our aid in a remarkable way in the question of diagnosis. The same may be said of the ethnic characteristics, especially the Mongolian type, which is so significant of congenital mental incapacity. In the developmental class I have already referred to the prow-shaped frontal bone as being highly typical and an aid to diagnosis, certainly helping us to assign a case to this division where there are psychological grounds for apprehending mental deficiency. With regard to the accidental class, physical deviations do not come to our aid. They have usually none of the grave deviations of conformation which we meet with in the congenital class. They have, as I have said, nothing in their look which would indicate their mental decadence. On the contrary, they in most cases during their childhood present physical features but little indicative of the terrible disaster which has befallen them; except in the paralysed sub-class they are fleet and mobile, and mischievous to a degree. They are irritated by constraint, are intolerant of having their heads examined, and try to escape from one's ken, they pull open every drawer that is unlocked, shake the handle of the room door to procure its opening, and sweep with their hand the ornaments off one's table that they may enjoy the rattle. They alternate their mischievous pranks with shrill and unmeaning cries. They rarely speak, are fond of feeling things with their tongues, and run about to get some fresh object on which to indulge this freak. They too frequently return a proferred kiss by a bite, and fill up the intervals of their mobile mischievousness by blowing bubbles with saliva on their lips. They have this important diagnostic feature, that they live entirely in a world of their own; they do not listen with a childlike curiosity to the conversation which is going on in their presence,—a conversation which is all-important to them, and in the outcome of which they are the most interested parties. They hear what is said, but they do not attend, nor can their attention be arrested, except by diverting them into new channels by a more attractive trail. They have usually great intensity of purpose, and succeed in having their own way, the mothers giving up the contest for the sake of peace. Slavering is a very common sign among the members of the three classes, arising sometimes from inattention, or from hyperæmic condition of the salivary glands, from prognathous form of jaw and inadequate size, or want of muscular power of lip, from inco-ordinate movements of the tongue, and sometimes from a combination of two or more of these conditions. Automatic movements are also very common; these may consist of rotatory movements of the head on its axis, of the body from side to side, or from back to front, or rhythmical movements of the fingers before the eyes.

There are a large number of boys and girls who are dull and backward and who develop tardily, but do arrive at last at a fair amount of intellectual power. They are the *enfants arrières* of the French writers. It is very important that their condition should be differentiated from that of idiots. Their state gives rise to much solicitude, and the prognosis depends very much on a right appreciation of their condition, as they respond very much to proper training. The test which I have found most useful is one suggested in the first instance by Dr. Charles West. In any given case we have to ask ourselves,—Can we in imagination put back the age two or more years and arrive thus at a time perfectly consistent with the mental condition of our patient? If he be a backward child we shall have no difficulty in saying what period of life would be in harmony with his state. If, however, he be an idiot there is no amount of imaginary antedated age to which the present condition of the child corresponds.

I have already referred to the frequency with

which lesions of speech occur among the feeble-minded. They often constitute a basis of great interest and importance for a diagnosis. The absence of speech when a child arrives at five or six years of age is in itself a matter for grave anxiety. It will be usually possible to refer the condition to one of three causes : (1) The child is completely deaf or has some slight congenital defect of hearing; or (2) there is some defect of conformation in the tongue, palate, or lips which prevents language being acquired; or (3) the child is defective in mental power, and either does not require speech from the absence of ideas or has an inability to convert ideas into words. Even when speech does exist it is often echo-like. I have had several children under my observation, in whom this kind of talking is characteristic—To my question, " How are you to-day ? " came the immediate reply, " To-day." I ask another, " Are you a good girl ? " the response is simply " Girl." Many such cases, however, may be gradually led to intelligent response. Sometimes the whole question is repeated, and the echo is not simply that of the last word. Often the absence of speech is associated with a perfect understanding of what is said, the speech faculty being a later development than the capacity for understanding spoken words. Gesture language frequently takes the place of spoken language in the feeble-minded. The want of speech is scarcely ever recognised by friends or relations as the outcome of feeble-mindededness. "My child," says almost invariably the mother or father, "has no deficiency except that he does not talk." When the child is being trained the parents regard the acquisition of, or improvement in, speech as the touchstone of progress, disregarding a number of other faculties which have been developed, or evil propensities which have been effaced. In many cases they are right, the absence of speech without deafness or deformity being a very important indication of a grave mental lesion.

A fertile field for the investigation of the morbid anatomy of idiocy is opened up by the enquiries of Hitzig, Jackson, and Ferrier into the localisation of function, and by improved microscopy aided by the use of staining agents. A very prominent characteristic is the diminished weight of the encephalon. Sometimes the diminution is very great, as in the microcephalic or Aztec variety. I have had the opportunity of examining several, but the most complete example was the brother of the boy described by Professor Marshall in the 'Transactions' of the Royal Society. The brother in question was for some years under my care, and was an extremely good example of the susceptibility to education of even most unpromising cases. He acquired language, read books with simple words, amused himself with pictures, and much enjoyed life. He was very agile, but always rested himself by placing his hands upon his knees, and when he ran he did so with his head far in advance of his body in a simian-like manner. He had a copious gesture language, which he had adopted before he acquired speech, and when he spoke he opened and shut his eyes and shook his head in a manner very suggestive of one of the quadrumana. He died at the age of eighteen. His mother had only given birth to two children, and they were both, as I have said, microcephalic. There was a history of extreme alcoholic intemperance on the part of the father, who died prematurely therefrom. The boy was 56 inches in height and weighed only 39 lbs. He died from phthisis with caseous deposit in his lungs and with more recent disseminated tubercle.

His head measured 15 inches in circumference. Its antero-posterior curve was 8 inches. Its bilateral curve 8 inches. Its antero-posterior diameter 5 inches, and its bilateral diameter 3·9 inches. The encephalon with its membranes weighed 15 ounces. The cerebrum was 4·2 inches long, 3·9 inches wide, and 1·8 inches high. It was attenuated in the occipital region in length, width and depth.

The departure from the ordinary course of development arose in all probability at an early period in the history of the germ. The convolutions which were best developed were those of the frontal, parietal, and temporal regions, while those less so were the orbital, but especially the occipital region. The central lobe, or Island of Reil, was represented only by a slightly elevated prominence. Gratiolet laid great stress on the supra-marginal lobule as characteristic of man; in this brain, however, the whole was reduced to the smallest possible size, while the bent fold was disproportionately large. Certainly the conformation is not explicable by reference merely to retarded growth, and lends, therefore, no countenance to the arguments of those who regard microcephalic brains as due simply to synostosis. In this case the sutures of the cranium remained with remarkable distinctness. The defect was one of development, and not of growth merely. The evidence of this is derived from the modification of the cerebral convolutions and the simplicity of their form. While all the parts of the perfect human cerebrum were represented, they, in a large number of cases, rivalled in simplicity the quadrumanous type. Like the brain described by Professor Marshall, the simplicity of arrangement was not equal throughout the whole of the convolutions, and here again some additional proof was offered of the arrest in development not having taken place at a definite period of embryonic existence.

On comparing this brain with that of his brother, it was noticed that while the parietal region remained the same, the frontal exceeded it in size. How far this was the result of the physical training to which he had been submitted one can only surmise. Certain it is that it is the only part of the brain which was proportionately larger than that of his brother, while the occipital lobe appeared to have undergone but little developmental change. Comparing his convolutions with those of the orang and chimpanzee they appeared to be less complex, the convolutions being smoother and less disturbed by secondary sulci. The absence of a well-defined supra-marginal lobule, the absence of the second connecting convolution, the simplicity of the bent convolution, the presence of the calcarine lobule, the absence of the accessory fold which unites the lobule of the second ascending fold to the superior marginal lobule, were all characters which approximated it to the quadrumanous brain. On the other hand, the want of symmetry, the presence of several of the external connecting folds, the absence of an operculum, the position from which the bent fold took its rise in reference to the fissure of Sylvius, the complete absence of the two internal connecting convolutions, and, lastly, the complete junction between the calloso-marginal and the middle temporal or uncinate convolutions were characters essentially human.

Cases of extreme asymmetrically developed brains are not infrequent; a very characteristic example I published in vol. xx of the "Pathological Transactions,' and many similar ones have come under my observation. The most frequent want of development is that of the occipital lobe. Where there is any approach to smallness of the brain this lobe is the part which shows greatest want of development. This condition has been noted in a case reported by Dr. Shuttleworth, in which the frontal and parietal lobes were fairly well developed but the occipital lobe was quite rudimentary. Dr. Fletcher Beach has also published some cases of microcephalism where the defective development of the occipital lobe was very marked.

Hypertrophy of the brain is not infrequently met with. In one very remarkable case that came under my observation there was the co-existence of a huge cranium with all the sutures completely ossified. So thoroughly was this the case that if it had occurred with a microcephalic cranium it would have been a strong argument in favour of the causal influence of premature synostosis in microcephalism. In another case the cranium was remarkably and uniformly thickened, and the brain weighed sixty-two ounces. On removing the dura mater the entire surface of the encephalon presented a blanc-mange appearance, in great measure obscuring the outline of the convolutions, which had great simplicity. The opacity appeared to be due to the presence of lymph, in the subarachnoid space, in the meshes of which lymph, limpid serum was contained. The substance of the brain was very tough and the cineritious portion pale. The subject was only fifteen years of age, and was remarkably stolid and irresponsive to all external impressions. Dr. Fletcher Beach has published a collection of cases which well illustrate hypertrophic conditions of the brain.

Absence, more or less complete, of the commissures is met with. In 2 per cent. of the cases I have examined there has been almost entire absence of the corpus callosum, and in 8 per cent. absence of the soft commissure.

Pallor of the grey portion of the encephalon is very frequently met with in the brains of feeble-minded children. Looking back over my post-mortem notes, nothing is more striking than the frequency with which extreme pallor is mentioned. I cannot but think that this affords indications for treatment as well as a basis for hopefulness in the possible functional improvement of the cerebrum.

The treatment of the various phases of feeble-mindedness resolves itself into medical and physical; and training, both moral and intellectual. The importance of commencing this betimes cannot be too much insisted on. Early training is of importance in preventing the growth of bad habits which become engrafted on the child. Constantly one meets with children who grow up a trouble to themselves and to those around them, from the injudicious treatment of some ignorant nurse who tyrannises over the family by her supposed essential relation to the child. Much time is often required to undo the evil—even if it be capable of being counteracted.

There are two great hindrances to the early and successful training of feeble-minded children arising from misconceptions on the part of many members of the medical profession. It is constantly said to the anxious parents of these children, "Do not be troubled, the child will grow out of it; wait till he reaches seven years," or, if the child has reached that age, then wait till he has reached fourteen. I know nothing of cataclysmal improvements, such as are here indicated. The opinion and advice have no bases in experience. The septennial periods referred to are periods of anxiety and peril; they are not periods of sudden leaps from mental feebleness to mental vigour; they are, on the contrary, developmental crises full of danger, periods when wreck of what mental power exists is liable to take place. How often one has cause to lament the precious time lost by the parents being thus lured into a fool's paradise! It should be remembered that the increments of intelligence are slow; that every proper habit has to be implanted; that many things which are thought instinctive and appear to come naturally, have, with painstaking solicitude, to be taught. Bad habits of the most serious kind spring up which militate against the progress of the child while waiting for the sudden change which never comes.

The other great mistake in the medical advice which is often given is the insistance to the mother that her child should not mix or be trained with children like himself, but with more intelligent children. Now, flattering as this may be to the parents, it is thoroughly baneful to the interest of the feeble-minded little one. The most successful training is effected with the child's equals; in this way a healthy emulation is established. Intelligent children will not take part in the amusements and games of feeble-minded ones, moreover, there is no community of feeling or of interest. The outcome of an attempt to train the feeble-minded child with others more intelligent than himself is infallibly to make his life *solitary* and to accentuate the condition which it is of the greatest importance to correct. I have seen the relative of a nobleman, living in all the luxury of a well-appointed country house, so put aside by her sisters, junior as well as senior, that she never ventured on a remark, and at length lost speech. I have seen the same girl transferred to a class of children like herself, pass from monosyllables to thorough conversational language, amid the sympathy and companionship of her compeers. Mothers of feeble-minded children invariably think their children more intelligent than any others of a like category, and they only need the bias of medical opinion to put off proper and effective aid until it is too late. Being afraid of their association with others of the same class, the parents either send them to schools where their lives are made wretched by teasing, and where they fall hopelessly behind, without the benefit of individual skill, or the helpfulness of collective emulation; or the boy is relegated to a country vicarage or Welsh farm, without any of the appliances or agencies which can develop his best possibilities. The first thing to be done is to rescue the feeble one from this *solitary* life, to give him suitable companionship, to place him in a condition where all the machinery shall move for his benefit, and where he shall be surrounded by influences of art and nature calculated to make his life joyous, to arouse his observation, and quicken his power of thought. No one who can speak from experience in the matter would hesitate in saying that the companionship of their equals in intellectual power provides just the attrition which is desirable,—that the association with their superiors condemns them to a life of isolation which renders nugatory all efforts for their improvement. The fear that the association of a feeble-minded child with feeble-minded children will exercise an injurious effect upon the growth of his intelligence is incorrect and not based upon experience.

Dr. Ireland has very well said that "imbecile children are no more injured by the presence of others of inferior intelligence than ordinary boys and girls are made childish by the appearance of a baby in the house,—that it is often, indeed, a great advantage for children to get rid of the uniform and hopeless inferiority in which they have hitherto lived, and to find that they have equals with whom they can interchange their simple ideas, and who give them a ready sympathy, and even to find that they have inferiors." How well I remember one feeble-minded boy coming to me and expressing his interest for another who was crippled, and saying to me, " Doctor, what a pity it is that that boy is lame, although he is not quite right." If there was any effect from the association it was that it begat a pharisaical spirit rather than exercised a depressing influence. The position of the feeble-minded is not always a very desirable one in the houses of the wealthy. Too often his claims are lost sight of, and the great aim is to keep his existence a secret, while no kind of companionship is established between him and the other members of the household. Moreover, the claims of society and the presence of visitors tend to make what little training there is desultory and futile, and lead to his being consigned to the care of servants in the less frequented portions of the house, where his life must necessarily be monotonous, uneventful, and uninteresting. If such are the difficulties among the wealthy, how much more are they intensified in the houses of the poor, where the parents are making a desperate struggle for existence,—where the afflicted little one uses up the time and energy of one sane life! How can it be possible, with the arrangements of a cottage, that anything tangible can be done to rescue the child from a condition which is deplorable in every aspect? Is it not probable that the mother, with her attention always directed to this object of care and anxiety, will propagate a neurotic race? Those who have witnessed the transformation in children who have been removed from squalid cottages to a well-regulated institution, or have seen their joyous return from luxurious homes to their companions and their training, will be able to realise how truthful is a mother's account of her boy that: "When putting him to bed the last night he was here he was smiles all over, saying, 'Going back to school to-morrow, mother,' and he packed his own bag before I could get to him in the morning, and could hardly finish breakfast he was in such a hurry to be off, and went away all smiles and delight."

It must always be kept in mind that the basis of all treatment should be *medical*. Medical, I mean, in an enlarged sense. Success can only be secured by maintaining the patient in the highest possible health. This is very well indicated by the intellectual torpor which follows or accompanies declension of health, and the lessened intellectual vigour which is met with in cold weather. I have referred to the hibernation which occurs among many feeble-minded children, and which has led me to notice that their intellectual vigour is *directly* as their external temperature. The pallor of the cineritious portions of their brains, which is so frequently met with, is suggestive of the necessity of vigorously maintaining their nutritive life. A very liberal dietary is of great importance. It should contain a fair quantity of nitrogenous elements, and be rich also in phosphatic and oleaginous constituents. Green vegetables are very essential, as in their absence there is a great tendency to become scorbutic. Care should be taken that farinaceous food, as represented by the so-called corn flours, should give way to the more plastic elements of nutrition found in semolina, entire wheat flour, or macaroni. Not only must the diet be sufficient in amount and good in quality, it should be exhibited in a form suited to their power of mastication. Their bedrooms and sitting-rooms should be spacious and well ventilated, and especially well warmed.

The skin should be kept in healthy function by frequent sponge and other baths, both for the sake of the individual health, and for the health and comfort of their associates. The exhalation from the skin of feeble minded children is something *sui generis*. It is of great importance that their residence should be on gravel soil, and with well-made walks, that no opportunity may be lost for outdoor exercise. Warm clothing is essential, to prevent as much as possible the disastrous effects of climatic changes. I have before referred to the relative frequency of phthisis to the ordinary mortality. Dr. Fitch, of Elwyn, Pennsylvania, in a very interesting paper, relates his experience that over 50 per cent. of his deaths were from disease of the lungs and air passages. My own experience is that on a clay soil 64 per cent., while on a gravel soil 44 per cent. of the mortality was from that cause. He also relates, what is in conformity with my experience, and in harmony with what I have been insisting on, that there is always a remarkable immunity from disease during the summer months. Having placed our patient under the most favorable hygienic conditions, the special training should be carried out with great enthusiasm. Physical training must form an important part of the education. The feeble muscles must be nourished by calling into exercise their functions, as well as by massage and by galvanism. Simple automatic movements, which I have referred to as being so common with the feeble-minded, should be replaced by others which are the product of will. We have to commence with very simple ones, gradually making them more complex. The want of co-ordination in the muscular system is very characteristic of the feeble-minded, and it is only by judicious physical training that the mutiny of the muscles can be overcome, and that purposeless acts can be converted into voluntary efforts suited for the wants of daily life. This training has to be carried out in great detail so that every voluntary muscle and every system of muscles may be called eventually into action. In this way the various acts of prehension, locomotion, and mastication are taught, the tongue becomes a willing agent, and the lips learn to retain the saliva which before gave our patient a repulsive look. I cannot enforce too strongly that little progress is made in speech until we first attain co-ordinated movements in the limbs. Finger lessons are to precede tongue lessons. I always remember the pinioned Frenchman who entreated that his arms might be freed because he wanted to speak. Unless we succeed in unpinioning the arms of our patients they do not speak. It is to be remembered too that we cannot bring into harmonious relation the muscles and the will without improving the physical quality of the brain and the other nervous centres. By these means, too, we shall have placed our patient in practical relation with the external world and initiated reasoning power.

The *moral* training is of great importance. While his physical and mental powers are being developed by hygienic and physiological processes, he has to be taught to subordinate his will to that of another. He has to learn obedience; that right-doing brings pleasure, and that wrong-doing is followed by its deprivation. The affective faculties should be so cultivated that the deprivation of the love of the teacher should be the greatest punishment and its manifestation the highest reward. In this way indications of untruthfulness, selfishness, obstinacy, sensuality, theft, and unkindness to companions are checked. Corporal punishment should be strictly forbidden. The tact of the teacher will be called into exercise in devising the suitable reward or punishment. I have seen a girl exhibiting violent obstinacy melted into contrition and obedience by the threat of the teacher that she would wipe from her face the kisses she had given her the previous day. In no case should the punishment interfere with the hygienic treatment. Nothing is worse than the deprivation of food for an offence. I have seen a case of violent and uncontrollable temper reduced to calm obedience by the administration of a basin of bread and milk. The moral delinquency was the result of mental excitement the outcome of defective nutrition.

The *intellectual* training must be based on a cultivation of the senses. They should be taught the qualities of form and the relation of objects by their sense of touch; to appreciate colour, size, shape, and relation by sight; to understand the varieties of sound when addressed to the ear; the qualities of objects by their taste and smell. The lessons should be of the simplest kind at first and gradually cumulative. Nothing is to be left to the imagination. The concrete must be taught, not the abstract. In this way we give them the basis from which their reasoning and reflective powers can be developed. Synchronously with this we make use of the physical powers we have cultivated. They should be taught to dress and undress. They should be trained to acquire habits of order and neatness, to use deftly the spoon or the knife and fork; to walk with precision and to handle with tact. The defective speech is best overcome by a well-arranged plan of tongue gymnastics, followed by a cultivation of the purely imitative powers, teaching at first monosyllabic sounds which have concrete representatives. The use and value of money where shops are not accessible is best taught by a plan I devised of instituting a shop furnished with the usual appliances of sale. One patient acted as the customer and another as the trader. In this way a purchase was effected and the whole transaction of buying, weighing, calculating, and paying, with the reception of change, was made under the criticism of the assembled class. All these belong to school instruction.

It is desirable, however, to supplement the house and school by gardening and farming operations ; by the lathe, the fretwork machine, the carpenter's bench, and, for the more advanced in education, the printer's shop. For girls, Kindergarten occupations and the various elegancies of needlework may be the outcome of persevering endeavours, while music and dancing may for all alternate with dramatic entertainments, which are most useful in appealing both to the eye and the ear. Care should be taken that the physical should interchange with the intellectual training. It is of the greatest importance that the teacher should keep clearly in view that his primary object is to make the pupil self-helpful, and, as far as possible, a useful member of the community; in this way more is done than by any other means. Mere *memoriter* knowledge is of little value; everything which makes him practically useful makes him proportionately happy.

But I am warned that my allotted time has expired. Methinks medicine of these later days, which has signalised her march by numerous victories, has had no more beneficent result than has been achieved by the enthusiasm of such men as Howe, Seguin, Wilbur, Knight, and Conolly of the past, and by those still living who are followers, it may be at a reverential distance, in the work of rescuing from oblivion and neglect a class who appeal to our tenderest sympathies and our most affectionate regards.

ACCOUNT OF A CASE

IN WHICH THE

CORPUS CALLOSUM AND FORNIX
WERE IMPERFECTLY FORMED

AND THE

SEPTUM LUCIDUM AND COMMISSURA
WERE ABSENT.

'Trans. of Roy. Med. and Chir. Soc.,' 1861.

THE medical literature of examples of defective commissures of the brain comprises so few cases, and of these the life-history is so imperfect, that I need no apology in placing the records of another before the members of this Society. The question has often been proposed to me, what relation idiocy bears to these arrests of development. At an early stage of my inquiry into the pathology of idiocy, I was prepared to meet with many cases characterised by the heading of this paper, but on further investigation found that, with the exception of deficient commissura mollis, absence or defect of the larger commissures of the brain occurred but seldom. Among fifty brains of idiots which I have dissected, the following is the only example of this nature.

That idiocy *frequently* depends on defective commissural connection my present experience does not support; but, on the other hand, that the absence of such connection may not *occasionally* be a cause of this calamity is, I apprehend, a question *sub judice*.

Mr. Paget, in the twenty-ninth volume of your 'Transactions,' has so ably generalised on the cases at that time on record, that there is little to be done beyond adding to the facts illustrating this interesting subject.

The case to which I beg leave to call your attention, is that of A. B—, a boy aged nine years at the time of his death. He had previously been under my daily observation for two and a half years. He was the first-born of three children; the second, a boy, is also idiotic; while the third and youngest, a girl, is healthy and intelligent. The respective ages of his father and mother, at the time of his birth, were twenty-six and twenty-seven years;

there was no consanguinity between them. There is no history of mental disease, or of any such defects as club-foot, hare-lip, cleft palate, &c., in either branch of the family. The mother's brother died of phthisis, but it was not thought to be owing in any way to constitutional predisposition. The mother, anteriorly to her marriage, had suffered intense pain in the left side, accompanied by hysteria; subsequently to her marriage, and during the pregnancy which speedily followed, there was no diminution, but rather an increase, of these sufferings. The pregnancy was attended by violent vomiting; and the pain in the side becoming more and more insupportable, opiates were largely resorted to for its relief. About this time Sir Benjamin Brodie was consulted, and his written opinion expresses the belief that she was suffering from renal oxalate-of-lime calculus. There were no unusual circumstances during parturition.

At five years of age the boy was received into the Asylum for Idiots at Earlswood. He was then a fair and delicate child, three feet three inches in height, fifty-three pounds and a half in weight; the shape of his head was oval, the circumference above the eyebrows eighteen inches and five eighths, length between the eyebrows and occipital protuberance eleven inches and three quarters, width of forehead four inches and a half. At this time he could stand alone, but was unable to walk; he was fed with a spoon, as he had no notion of masticating, and it was necessary for his nurse to convey the food to the fauces in order to excite the reflex act of deglutition. He could not speak, and was very spiteful. His habits were dirty, and this was augmented by frequent diarrhœa. When seven years old he was able to walk, though feebly, and was placed in the infant class for training and instruction. At nine, the period of his death, he could walk and run, his spiteful habits had been overcome, he was mild and tractable, and exhibited much fondness for his younger brother. He was timid, and afraid of certain toys, did not play with other children, and found most amusement in looking at a picture scrap-book. He was fond of listening to music; had little or no power of imitation. Although great pains were taken to instruct him, he could scarcely be said to have learned anything. He would in some measure go through simple exercises in drilling at command, but could not be taught to throw a ball with any aim. There was no want of co-ordination in his movements, and no diminution of sensation; his habits had become moderately correct; he was able to feed himself with a spoon, the meat having been previously minced, and with much difficulty he was taught to raise a cup to his mouth. He remembered his father and mother; on seeing any lady in black, the colour usually worn by his mother, he would approach, and after examination would say, " No, mamma ! no !" which, with the word " *me* " when he wanted anything, was the full extent of his powers of utterance. He had no vivacity, and his extreme pallor was remarkable.

His physical health was far from good; he was never long free from either strumous ophthalmia, eruptions at the nasal and oral orifices, thecal abscesses, or diarrhœa; but he had never been subject to convulsions or epileptic fits. He died from pneumonia on the right side.

A post-mortem examination was made thirty-three hours after death. The right lung was hepatized throughout, except at its anterior margin. Several of Peyer's glands in the ileum were enlarged and congested. The large intestine extremely congested throughout. The testes had descended into the scrotum, but were small; the pubes was sparsely covered with hair. The other organs were healthy.

The calvarium was of normal thickness, but somewhat unsymmetrical; there were granular patches in the arachnoid on both sides of the longitudinal fissure, and between these and the dura mater slight adhesions. The encephalon weighed two pounds eight ounces avoirdupois; the cavity of the arachnoid contained about two ounces of straw-coloured serum; the membranes and sinuses normal. The antero-posterior diameter of the cerebrum was six and a half, its width five and a half inches; the width of each hemisphere measured across the anterior lobe, in front of the remnant of the corpus callosum, two and a quarter inches. The antero-posterior diameter of each hemisphere of the cerebellum was two and a quarter, its entire width three and a half inches.

On making sections of the cerebrum and cerebellum, there was nothing noticeable respecting the size, form, arrangement, or colour of the convolutions. On the first removal of the encephalon from the cranium, it was noticed that, on being placed in its natural position, the hemispheres separated to an unusual extent, without bringing into view the great commissure of the brain, but displaying, instead, the velum interpositum. Anterior to the velum, and on the same plane, was exposed, on forcibly separating the hemispheres, a narrow band of medullary structure. A horizontal section of both hemispheres, so as to display the interior of the lateral ventricles, was then made, and the velum interpositum removed. The brain was in no part of its structure deficient in cohesion; the posterior cornu of each of the lateral ventricles was enlarged, and contained about half an ounce of straw-coloured serum each. The small hippocampus on each side was rather large; the tænia semicircularis very fully developed. At this stage of the dissection no remnant of the fornix could be discerned; there was positive absence of any septum lucidum. The third ventricle was exposed, but no middle commissure could be discovered; the pineal gland occupied its usual position between the lobes of the corpora quadrigemina, all which structures were of normal size and appearance. At the anterior boundary of the third ventricle there was the before-mentioned medullary band, which was regarded as the representative of the corpus callosum, but occupying a much lower plane than the normal position of the commissure. It presented, both anteriorly and posteriorly, crescentic, thinned margins, and measured at its narrowest part, which was slightly to the left of the mesial line, one third of an inch. A section was then made through both hemispheres on a level with the transverse band. The optic thalami were unusually flattened, and their inner surfaces indicated that the soft commissure had never been present. There was a marked absence of the peduncles of the pineal gland. The third ventricle presented on its floor the usual structures, and at its anterior part could now be seen the anterior pillars of the fornix ascending at slight angles, but widely separated throughout. Beneath the posterior margin of the transverse band they made a sudden bend, and, passing outward and backward over the upper surface of the optic thalami, terminated in the descending cornua of the lateral ventricles as the tæniæ hippocampi, the tæniæ, however, being narrower than usual.

The optic commissure at the floor of the third ventricle was strongly marked, and the lamina cinerea interleaved between it and the anterior commissure, where it terminated. The anterior commissure was well defined, and above it an interval of two lines occurred between it and the transverse band. The inner surfaces of the anterior lobes of the cerebrum were separated inferiorly as far as the anterior commissure; and the parts of them into which the knee and reflected portion or rostrum of the corpus callosum are usually inserted were covered with convolutions such as are common to other parts of the cerebral surface. The band or rudiment of corpus callosum was situated opposite the widest portion of the corpora striata; its anterior edge being two and one twelfth inches from the anterior margin of the cerebral hemispheres, and its posterior border being four and one twelfth inches from the posterior margin of the hemispheres. It did not exceed one sixteenth of an inch in thickness at any part of it, and its fibres spread out anteriorly and posteriorly on reaching the hemispheres. It will follow from this description that there was no representative of the genu or of the reflexed portion of the corpus callosum; that the body of the fornix, septum lucidum, and its fifth ventricle, and the soft or middle commissure, were entirely absent; and that there existed no communication between the lateral representatives of the fornix; moreover, that these had no connection with the posterior diverging fibres of the transverse band, and consequently that not even the analogue of a septum lucidum was present.

Mr. Paget, in the twenty-ninth volume of your 'Transactions,' has grouped together with his own case others related by Reil, Mr. Solly, and Mr. Chatto, and has made some important physiological deductions. The case related by him was "not remarkable for any excellence or great defect of mind." In Mr. Solly's, the boy, although "boobyfied," could read, and selected as his favourite reading religious books. Reil's case, a woman, was of dull intellect, but could go errands in the village. Mr. Chatto's patient lived only twelve months.

In comparing the case which has been here detailed with those referred to by Mr. Paget, it would, at first sight, appear to stand opposed to the conclusions at which he arrived, and to support the view that the corpus callosum is necessary to the possession of the average power of the human mind. But this opposition may be *only* apparent; for it is a circumstance worthy of special regard in instituting a comparison, that while in the three above-named examples the soft commissure was present, in the one which I have brought forward it was entirely absent. Moreover, in Mr. Solly's case, the soft commissure was " wide and thick," and in Mr. Paget's it was inordinately large, measuring six tenths of an inch from before backwards, and being also thicker than usual.

How far the presence of extra large, middle commissures compensated for other deficiencies in the former cases, and how far its absence was the cause of the extreme mental deficiency in the present instance, I shall not now discuss. I will only say that my researches hitherto lead me to attach a physiological importance to the soft commissure which previous observers have not recorded.

ON THE

CONDITION OF THE MOUTH IN IDIOCY.

The 'Lancet,' vol. i, 1862.

The opinion which has been formed, both in and out of the profession, in reference to idiocy, has arisen more from the representations of poets and romance-writers than from the deductions of rigid observation. The popular novelist, in this as in other cases, seizes on the characteristics of some exaggerated specimen, pourtrays them by the aid of a vivid imagination, and henceforth the exaggeration becomes the type of a species in the minds of men. The term idiot has thus become synonymous with the most degraded condition of humanity only —with a creature incapable of being influenced by moral or physical treatment, and separated by an immense gulf from the remainder of mankind. It has arisen, in no small degree, from the existence of this opinion, that until within a comparatively recent period, so few efforts have been made to ameliorate the condition of idiots. In too many cases they have been neglected or allowed to be influenced for evil, regardless of the fact that they might be equally impressed for good. Independently of the benefit that can be effected for these unfortunate sufferers, the benevolent efforts on their behalf have furnished an opportunity for an investigation into their physical and psychical life before unattainable.

The condition of the idiot is not simply one of mental alienation. It frequently presents also grave physical deterioration; and this physical alteration is as much a test of idiocy as is the low condition of mental power. In a community such as that of the Earlswood Asylum, there is to be found every variety of imbecile mind. In fact, just as in the outer world there is a graduated series from the most commonplace intellects,—who are " the hewers of wood and drawers of water,"—up to the giant minds that leave their impress on the age in which they live; so is there amongst an imbecile population a gradual shading in an inverse direction—from the youth who might, if he had property, become the subject of inquiry before a Master in Lunacy, to one who, with every means of communication with the external world, except feeling, closed, vegetates in impenetrable mist. In such a community one can perceive the grades of physical condition accompanying the mental phases; and a study of the physical anomalies becomes as interesting and important as that of the psychological state. When contemplating so large a number as that which Earlswood shelters, one is able to set some of the members aside into natural groups, by simple reference to their physical state, and to predicate from that state what will be their probable future mental improvement.

There is scarcely an organ in the body but may be found gravely altered in idiots: the circulation and respiration are abnormal; the skin exhibits perturbed functions; defective innervation, lesions of motility and nutrition, are abundantly met with; the bodily conformation is often of an aberrant kind. Regard therefore should be paid, in all cases of diagnosis of idiocy, to the physical condition as confirmatory of any opinion based on purely psychological data. It is in this way one is enabled to differentiate an idiot from a simply backward or ill-regulated child.

It is from the conviction of the importance of a study of the physiological manifestations of idiocy, that I have been induced to devote no small portion of time to an investigation into the structure and functions of the various organs *seriatim* amongst idiots and imbeciles. I purpose in the present paper giving some of the results of my observations of the feeble-minded, in reference to the condition and conformation of their mouths. Characteristic as is this region of various transitory mental phases amongst the sane, does it bear the permanent impress of a state in which the mind has failed in attaining its normal condition? If so, what is the nature of the impress? Does any value attach to the conformation of the mouth as confirmatory or otherwise of a state of mental incapacity? These are some of the questions we have to solve.

I may premise that these observations have been made during the past year, without reference to any recent legal inquiry, and extend over 200 cases, which have been taken, without any special selection, from a larger number. Not one on the list would in his present condition be able to manage his own affairs, or be legally held to be responsible. Many of them, however, are susceptible of considerable culture, are affected by the amenities of life, write letters to their friends, make small purchases, and form friendships. Several perform mechanical work with system and order. One, although possessing very little judgment, has been taught French and Latin, and reads these languages as well as ordinary schoolboys. Some few possess extraordinary memories and special aptitudes. 146 were males, and 54 females. Their ages ranged from seven to thirty-six, and the following table gives the numbers at each age last birthday :—

No.	Age.	No.	Age.	No.	Age.
2 at 7	...	14 at 16	...	5 at 25	
4 ,, 8	...	18 ,, 17	...	1 ,, 26	
2 ,, 9	...	10 ,, 18	...	3 ,, 27	
4 ,, 10		14 ,, 19		2 ,, 28	
10 ,, 11		18 ,, 20		1 ,, 29	
13 ,, 12	...	7 ,, 21	...	3 ,, 30	
11 ,, 13	...	12 ,, 22	...	2 ,, 33	
12 ,, 14	...	9 ,, 23		1 ,, 34	
17 ,, 15		3 ,, 24		2 ,, 36	

Or ranged in decennial periods—below 10 years, 8; from 10 to 19 inclusive, 123; from 20 to 29, 61; from 30 to 39, 8.

Palate.—Amongst the 200 cases included in this inquiry, 82 possessed palates inordinately arched, and with this increased arching were noticed various abnormalities. In some the palate was unsymmetrical, the two sides having different degrees of concavity, or one side plane, and the other concave. In 34 the palates were excessively arched, approximating to the appearance of the roof of a house, and, with this extreme angularity, was great narrowness. Excessive arching of the palate occurred, therefore, in 58 per cent. Excessive flattening of the palate was observed in 4 cases. In 34 cases, or 17 per cent., the palate had a very prominent antero-posterior ridge or keel, corresponding to the line of approximation of the palatal bones. In 7 the palate bones did not meet, leaving a sulcus between them, the mucous membrane being, however, continuous. There was no instance of the ordinary cleft palate, and I may remark that in an examination of nearly 600 idiots, I have failed in meeting with an example of that deformity. In several the hard palate extended but a short distance posteriorly, from defect of the palatal process of the superior maxillary bone and entire absence of the palatal process of the palate bone, and in all these cases the velum palati was unusually flaccid. In the majority of cases there was marked narrowness of the palate. The following table represents the measurements in 24ths of an inch of the space between the posterior bicuspid teeth of opposite sides :—

No.	Distance. In.	No.	Distance. In.	No.	Distance. In.
2	at $\frac{16}{24}$	11	at $\frac{23}{24}$	13	at $1\frac{5}{24}$
1	,, $\frac{18}{24}$	24	,, 1	9	,, $1\frac{6}{24}$
3	,, $\frac{19}{24}$	37	,, $1\frac{1}{24}$	1	,, $1\frac{7}{24}$
2	,, $\frac{20}{24}$	25	,, $1\frac{2}{24}$	5	,, $1\frac{8}{24}$
13	,, $\frac{21}{24}$	23	,, $1\frac{3}{24}$	3	,, $1\frac{12}{24}$
10	,, $\frac{22}{24}$	17	,, $1\frac{4}{24}$	1	,, $1\frac{22}{24}$

It will be observed that 33 per cent. do not exceed 1 inch, and that 62 per cent., while being more than 1 inch, do not exceed $1\frac{1}{4}$ inch; whereas the normal average has been stated to be $1\frac{1}{2}$ inch. It is worthy of notice that these numbers hold no direct relation to the age or stature of the patients examined. Thus, in a youth 22 years of age and 6 ft. 1 in. in height, so narrow is the palate that there is only $1\frac{2}{24}$ inch between the bicuspids, and only $\frac{10}{24}$ inch between the opposite gums at their widest interval. The lowest measurements occurred in a boy and girl, the boy 12 and the girl 13 years of age. Neither is there a direct relation between the width of the palate and the cranial capacity; for in a microcephal, whose palate was $\frac{22}{24}$ inch wide, the internal canthi of the eyes were $\frac{23}{24}$ inch distant from one another; while in a macrocephal whose palate was $\frac{23}{24}$ inch wide, the distance between the internal canthi amounted to 2 inches.

Teeth.—The principal characteristics of the teeth in idiots are, that the period of the first dentition is delayed, the second dentition considerably postponed, and that they undergo very general and rapid decay. In many cases the anterior surface of the incisors presents a honeycombed appearance, but in no one instance have I observed those special characters which have been well shown by Mr. Hutchinson to be significant of congenital syphilis. In a large number of cases they are developed irregularly, are crowded, and the canine occupy a different plane from the other teeth,—all these irregularities resulting from the imperfect development of the superior maxillary bone. In 6 cases, or 3 per cent., the upper incisors projected to such an extreme degree as to produce grave deformity. In 7 cases the teeth of the lower jaw were in advance of those of the upper.

Tongue.—The most prevailing character noticeable in the tongue of idiots is the hypertrophy of the fungiform papillæ. Undue prominence of the papillæ was observed in 101 instances. In several there is a marked want of co-ordination in the movements of the tongue, so that the patient, although endeavouring to comply with the request, is unable to protrude it. This condition is usually associated with an absence of general co-ordinated movements, and in the improvement which is effected by treatment it is usually the most persistent derangement of motility. In 16 cases the tongue presented a soddened appearance and exhibited deep transverse furrows on its dorsal surface; in all these patients one is able to trace a marked physiological and psychological agreement, and so much do they resemble one another in these respects that they might readily be taken for members of the same family. Inordinate size occurred in 12 instances, and in almost every case was associated with defective power of articulation. In 2 the tongue was unusually long; 33 were mute; 16 semi-mute. In 83 the speech was indistinct. In 62 the speech was fair. Stammering was observed in 4.

Tonsils.—One cause of the peculiar speech prevailing among idiots is the condition of the tonsils. These observations for the most part were made in the summer, when the tonsils were not likely to be rendered worse than their usual condition by climatic influences. In 30 instances they were injected, in 17 slightly enlarged, in 79 considerably enlarged, and in 5 so much increased in size as to interfere with deglutition and respiration.

Mucous membrane, &c.—Besides the injection of the mucous membrane of the tonsils which has been noticed, other regions of the oral cavity are liable to this condition. The velum palati, uvula, and pillars of the pharynx were found to be thus characterised in 27 instances. The posterior wall of the pharynx was observed to be marked by considerable vascular injection in 33 cases, and in 6 the mucous membrane had assumed a granular appearance. The buccal and labial glands were generally hypertrophied, and the salivary glands were frequently enlarged. In 11 instances the sublingual gland was *greatly* enlarged. The uvula was elongated in 14 cases, bifid in 2, very short in 1, and entirely absent in 1. The lips were hypertrophied in 2. Owing probably to the abundant supply of fresh vegetables with which the patients are provided, I only found one case in which the gums were swollen and tumid.

Slavering.—The flow of saliva from the mouth is universally associated in the popular mind with the condition of idiocy. The slavering may vary in degree. It may occur only at periods of excitement, and at meal times, or with scarcely any intermission throughout the day, producing in severe cases excoriation of the chin. Amongst 325 cases which I have examined, I find 72, or 22 per cent., in which this habit was noticed. Of these, 28 slaver to a slight extent, 17 rather more so, and 26 in an aggravated degree. This peculiarity depends, I believe, on two or three causes—1st, the increased secretion of saliva; 2nd, the deformed condition of the mouth; 3rd, the want of co-ordinated movements in the muscles of the tongue; and 4th, the absence of tonicity in the labial muscles. Seeing that slavering exists in 22 per cent. of imbeciles, the question may arise—Is it confined to this section of the community? I am not prepared to say that it is never associated with mental vigour; but I believe that, excluding childhood, old age, disease of the mouth and neural lesions, slavering is very rarely unconnected with mental imbecility. Moreover, I have examined with reference to this question 1000 persons, who are doing the everyday work of the world, without meeting with a single example.

Summary.—We have thus seen that idiocy is not simply a cerebral lesion; that it carries with it marked physical deviations, of which I have shown conspicuous examples in the mouth; narrowed, arched, and unsymmetrical palates; tardily developed, irregular, and rapidly decaying teeth; a hyperæmic condition of the mucous membrane and glands; elongated uvulas and hypertrophied tonsils; large, enervated, and rugous tongues, deficient in co-ordinated movements and in their special function; saliva secreted inordinately, and retained incontinently. Such are some of the characteristics of a class, in which mental vigour is in abeyance, which should be taken in connection with the psychological state in diagnosis, and inculcate the doctrine that the psychical condition of these unfortunates should be specially sought to be ameliorated by an improvement of their physical condition.

ON

POLYSARCIA AND ITS TREATMENT.

'London Hospital Reports,' 1864.

THE term polysarcia has been so long accepted as a designation of that condition of the body, in which the purely adipose constituents are developed in excess, that I am induced to employ it, although its literal significance is not strictly in accordance with the pathological state.

The history of Medicine contains numerous instances of extraordinary obesity, and an immortality attaches to some names, solely on account of special aptitude for the development of fat. It is not in reference to such exceptional examples as some of the earlier records of medicine unfold, that the practitioner is likely to be consulted, but the cases are not infrequent in which his aid may be solicited in mitigating the inconveniences which excessive adipose development entails.

The sufferers from this disease are found more frequently among those on whom fortune has smiled, whose incentives to physical exertion are in abeyance, while the inducements of the table are in excess. Nevertheless among the out-patients of the hospital, I have noticed several cases, in which polysarcia has been the cause of a variety of subjective symptoms which have made life wretched. The subjects have been for the most part women who had passed the climacteric period. They have resorted to the mental solace which alcoholic potations could afford, and their diet, though poor, has been of the kind calculated to induce this state.

Dr. Flemyng, in a paper read before the Royal Society in 1757, regarded corpulency as caused either by the introduction of too much oil in the food, or by the over-largeness of the cells, in which it is deposited—or by a crasis of the blood allowing the oily particles to be strained off too easily—or, lastly, by a deficient evacuation of oil already taken in and separated from the blood.

His remedies were addressed either to increasing the evacuation by the bowels, the sweat-glands, or the renal organs. Diuresis was his principal hope, inasmuch, he said, as "the animal oil is carried out of the body in the urine." The diuretic he selected was soap, from his supposing it to have the property of " besides increasing the quantity of urine, at the same time rendering the animal oil more mixible with the watery vehicle of the blood."

Darwin, in his 'Zoonomia,' recommends aerated alkaline water, from an idea of its rendering fat more fluid. Dr. Cullen was of opinion that "the diet must be sparing, or rather, what is more admissible, it must be such as affords little nutritious matter; it must, therefore," he said, "be chiefly or almost only of vegetable matter, and, at the very utmost, milk."

Dr. Brown argues "that as animal food is the principal noxious power, the quantity should be reduced, and more exercise taken."

Dr. Fothergill states that "a strict vegetable diet produces exuberant fat more certainly than any other means I know." He enjoins, moreover, "an abstinence from animal food, so far as the patient's health, situation, and manner of life, will admit of it." Dr. Bright has advised iodide of potassium with the view of giving tone to the absorbents. Alkalies, from their power of saponifying fats, and thus rendering them more miscible, have had their advocates.

More recently, Dr. Duchesne-Duparc has spoken highly of the effect of the extract of the fucus vesiculosus, stating that it increases the appetite, diuresis, and emaciation.

The following case of polysarcia, which has been for some time under my observation, has given me an opportunity of testing the value of some of these remedies which have been recommended, and of proving the superior efficacy of that which I believe to be the true physiological mode of treatment.

E. C—, a girl of healthy parentage, and born in the county of Norfolk, became an inmate of the Asylum for Idiots at Earlswood, in the year 1850, at the age of thirteen years. From notes taken by Dr. Foreman at the time of her admission, I learn that she was congenitally of feeble mind, was four feet four inches in height, and weighed in her clothes 113 lbs.; her size at that time attracted observation, as it is noted, " she is enormously stout, cellular tissue everywhere more than usual." Her diet was not much restricted, and she always appears to have been voracious in appetite. In January, 1857, Dr. Maxwell added to the above notes that she was still the same height, but weighed 151 lbs., and up to that time had not menstruated. She came under my treatment in November, 1858, when I found her indulging in a large mixed diet, with excess of vegetables, and taking very little exercise, and her size was steadily increasing. Her height was still the same, and her weight 196 lbs. Her unwieldy size rendered exercise difficult. From inquiries made of her friends, I found there had been no such instance of obesity among the relatives of her progenitors —that she had been delicate and thin up to seven years of age.

Her diet was restricted to the following scale, which was accurately weighed for each meal :— Breakfast, six ounces of bread; one third ounce of butter; half-pint of milk-and-water. Dinner—four ounces of meat (weighed, when cooked, and free from bone); eight ounces of potatoes; two ounces of green vegetables; six ounces of pudding; half-pint of water. Supper —six ounces of bread; one third ounce of butter; half-pint of milk-and-water. (The milk-

and-water was a mixture of one third new milk and two thirds water.) Walking exercise was enforced, and she was required to turn the handle of a large mincing-machine one hour a day.

My note-book states that in January, 1862, she remained the same height (four feet four inches), but had increased in weight. She was then 210 lbs. when weighed in her night-dress, and measured, round her waist, fifty-five inches. Her feet and hands remained small, and contrasted remarkably with the appendages they terminated. She had no hair in the axillæ, and scarcely any on the pubis. Although twenty-five years of age she had never menstruated, nor did she exhibit the slightest sexual instinct. She was now able to walk slowly, but with difficulty, and when she fell, was unable without assistance to regain the vertical position. She suffered from dyspnœa, and her breathing at night was attended by so much noise that the occupants of the same room were much disturbed thereby. Moreover, the difficulty she had in moving from her bed had induced dirty habits, which added much to the wretchedness of her life. It was now difficult to induce her to take any exercise, and she was scarcely seated in a chair for a minute without falling asleep. Although imbecile in mind, her obesity was a mental trouble to her, and she was ready to enter into any plan for diminishing her size.

Being desirous of ascertaining the effect of medication simply, the same diet was continued, and iodide of potassium, in doses of two and a half grains, given three times a day, for a period of six months, without any diminution of size. Her health continued unaltered. The only effect produced was a cessation of the development of fat, which had been constant for the past twelve years.

The diet remaining the same, solution of potash was given three times a day in doses of ten drops, gradually increased to half a drachm, over a period of seven months. Under this treatment her health became deteriorated, presenting symptoms of anæmia, and her weight oscillated around fifteen stone, sometimes a few pounds more, sometimes as many less.

When the alkali was discontinued, on February 13th, 1863, she weighed in her nightdress 206 lbs. A diminution was thus effected of 4 lbs. after seven months' exhibition of caustic potash. Still continuing the same mixed diet, the extract of fucus vesiculosus (prepared by Messrs. Rew and Co., of Regent Street) was given in doses of half a drachm three times a day until April 30th, when she weighed 203 lbs.

The effect of the fucus was to promote diuresis, as indicated by an increased number of wet beds, and a diminution of weight at the rate of four ounces and one third per week. Her general health had improved, and she was much less anæmic than when she discontinued the potash.

On April 30th, in conformity with a previously arranged plan, I discontinued all medicaments, and placed her on very rigid animal diet. Her breakfast consisted of five ounces of cold roast meat, free from fat, and half a pint of tea, with very little milk, and no sugar (no bread). Dinner—six ounces of hot roast meat, free from fat, two ounces green vegetables (no potatoes or bread), half a pint of water. Supper the same as breakfast. In order to induce her compliance, she had one ounce of sherry wine, and occasionally a baked apple with her dinner, and to prevent the possibility of her obtaining any food from others, strict supervision was exercised.

After she had been subjected to this diet for a week she had slight febrile disturbance, and for three days took one quart of beef-tea a day, made from one pound of beef. She then returned to her meat diet, which was continued without intermission until August 29th, when she weighed 175 lbs. The effect of this diet was to improve her general health and physical power. She was enabled to run, and she took walks with pleasure. The dyspnœa had disappeared, and her clothes had to be altered to suit her diminished form. Her loss of weight had been at the rate of one pound and three-quarters per week.

Wishing to ascertain whether the fucus vesiculosus would influence the system when a purely animal diet was used, half a drachm of the extract was now given three times a day, while the diet was restricted to sixteen ounces of meat. This was continued until November 14th, when she was attacked by scarlet fever; her weight had receded to 153 lbs., the diminution having been at the rate of one pound thirteen ounces one third per week, or one ounce one third per week more than when the meat was given without the fucus. During the attack of scarlet fever and the subsequent convalescence, the diet was beef-tea with bread; and on this diet, at the end of four weeks, her weight remained without alteration. On December 12th she returned to meat diet, substituting, however, fifteen ounces for sixteen ounces per diem. This has been continued to the present time (January 15th, 1864); her weight is now 147 lbs., and the measurement round the waist has diminished from fifty-five inches to thirty-seven inches. Her general health is good, and the restricted diet has not been attended by any inconvenience. The following tables will give, in a condensed form, the results:—

	Weekly Increase in weight.	Weekly Decrease in weight.
Mixed diet, unrestricted in amount	$7\frac{3}{4}$ oz.	
Mixed diet, restricted in amount	$1\frac{2}{5}$ oz.	
Mixed, restricted diet, and Iodide of Potassium	nil	nil.
Mixed, restricted diet, and Liquor Potassæ	—	$2\frac{1}{7}$ oz.
Mixed, restricted diet, and Fucus Vesiculosus	—	$4\frac{1}{3}$ oz.
Purely meat diet, without medicine	—	28 oz.
Purely meat diet, with Fucus Vesiculosus	—	$29\frac{1}{3}$ oz.

Date.	Age.	Weight.
28th Feb., 1850	13	113 lbs.
Jan., 1857	20	151 ,,
Nov., 1858	21½	196 ,,
Jan., 1862	25	210 ,,
13th Feb., 1863	26	206 ,,
30th April —	—	203 ,,
22nd Aug. —	26½	175 ,,
14th Nov. —	—	153 ,,
15th Jan., 1864	27	147 ,,

It is only by returning to the views and opinions of medical authorities a century ago that we can duly appreciate the vast service chemistry has rendered physiology, and, indirectly, practical medicine. The influence of respiration in removing carbonaceous materials from the blood, and the possibility of the production of fat from farinaceous and saccharine bodies, are so familiar to us that we wonder at the absence of knowledge on these subjects displayed by the older writers. They all insist on a non-nutritious diet for the cure of obesity, meaning thereby an expurgation of meat and an indulgence in milk and farina. A great mistake was also made in supposing that the urine was the outlet for fatty matters, while they ignored the outlet by the lungs.

On a review of the foregoing case, it is worthy of notice that the young woman has never menstruated, and this, together with the absence of sexual instinct, suggests the idea that the ovaries are undeveloped, and that she may be in the condition of a pig which has been spayed for the purpose of fattening. Her voracious appetite, and a diet in which farinaceous matters largely entered, were doubtless factors in the production of the result. When the diet, however, was restricted to the amount on which her companions were only fairly nourished, still she made fat in excess, to the amount of one ounce and two fifths per week.

The exhibition of iodide of potassium failed to be of value, other than preventing a continuation of the morbid increase, while liquor potassæ, by interfering with digestion and undermining her general health, produced slight positive diminution. The results obtained from the fucus vesiculosus were such as to justify its being regarded as a safe and, to a certain extent, effectual plan for diminishing obesity. It falls, however, far behind what it is possible to effect by a purely animal diet, and while to many the latter remedy may appear as bad as the disease, it should be remembered that a diet so purely animal need not be insisted upon, a compromise may be made, keeping in view the typical diet which should be approached as nearly as possible in the treatment of these cases.

It has been shown by Ranke that even when large quantities of meat are taken, a decrease in the weight of the body takes place, but that the quantity of meat theoretically requisite to maintain the system produces dyspepsia. In the treatment of polysarcia, this difficulty is avoided, the quantity of meat is regulated to supply the want induced by the tissue-changes of the body, trusting to the superabundant fatty matters of the system to supply the demand of the respiratory process. In the case I have detailed, the patient has continued the meat diet for nine months without any dyspepsia, with improved tone, with a power of resisting such a disease as scarlet fever, making a speedy convalescence therefrom, and with the positive advantages of diminished size and increased enjoyment of life.

April 7th.—The patient has continued on a diet of 15 oz. of meat daily, and her present weight is 133 lbs., indicating a continued diminution at the rate of one pound two ounces and a half a week. Her total loss in weight has been 77 lbs.; her decrease during the last year, 70 lbs.

AN ACCOUNT OF A SECOND CASE

IN WHICH THE

CORPUS CALLOSUM WAS DEFECTIVE.

'Trans. of Roy. Med. & Chir. Soc.,' 1866.

IN the forty-fourth volume of the 'Transactions' of this Society I furnished the details of a case in which there was a marked defect in the great commissural connections of the brain, associated with grave defect of the intellectual faculties. I, at the same time, compared the case under review with all others of a similar nature which I could find recorded.

Another instance having come under my notice which illustrates, in a characteristic way, this rare abnormality, I am desirous of placing it on record in the 'Transactions' of the same Society, which already contains descriptions of the best marked examples.

A. B. came under my observation in the

autumn of 1858. He was the son of a clergyman, and had been submitted to the ordinary process of education with but trifling results. He had been taught to write a little, but he never exercised the art. He had learned to read easy words, and could answer simple questions. His power of calculation was almost *nil*. He was fond of music, had slight power of imitation, and his memory, although defective, was good in relation to persons and things. He was five feet four and three quarter inches in height, and weighed ten stone one pound. His trunk was well formed, and his facial expression that of an imbecile. He was shy, undemonstrative, fond of children (some of whom he petted), while towards persons of his own age and to the opposite sex he was violent and passionate. His friends were very desirous of asserting the non-congenital nature of the mental condition, and attributed it to masturbation. The diagnosis formed, however, was that it was congenital, and that the masturbation was an accidental circumstance. This diagnosis was strengthened by reference to the other members of the family, who, although occupying good positions in the world, were manifestly not of average intellectual power. The habit of masturbation became entirely broken, and he gave himself up to simple employments, such as wheeling invalids in a Bath chair, and otherwise aiding those whom he petted.

He lived to forty years of age, when he died from pleuro-pneumonia. An autopsy was made thirty hours after death. The circumference of the head was $21\frac{1}{4}$ in.; the bilateral curve $11\frac{1}{2}$ in.; the antero-posterior curve 12 in.; the bilateral diameter $5\frac{8}{10}$ in.; the antero-posterior diameter $6\frac{7}{10}$ in. The calvarium was unsymmetrical and dense, shelving anteriorly; the posterior clinoid processes were converted into sharp needle-like points; the encephalon weighed 2 lb. 14 oz. On separating the two hemispheres the almost entire absence of the corpus callosum was apparent, and the velum interpositum exposed to view. A small cartilaginous-like band, $\frac{7}{24}$ in. in breadth and $\frac{1}{24}$ in. in thickness, situated opposite the corpora striata, was the only representative of the great commissure. The fornix was represented by two thin posterior pillars; the body of the fornix and its anterior pillars were absent.

The right optic thalamus was very much larger than the left. The cineritious portion of the brain was pale, the posterior cornua of the lateral ventricles were distended with straw-coloured serum, and the Pineal gland was the size of a wild cherry. The middle commissure was absent. The rarity of this abnormality may be indicated by the circumstance that it is only the second time I have met with it in the dissection of 150 brains of idiots.

MARRIAGES OF CONSANGUINITY

IN RELATION TO

DEGENERATION OF RACE.

'London Hospital Reports,' 1866.

PROBABLY no subject which has engaged the attention of the medical statist has given rise to more widely divergent views, certainly no inquiry on the part of the physiologist, has been productive of less practical results, than the one which heads this paper. There is a class, and probably a large one, which looks upon consanguineous unions as universally productive of evil, and where the worst consequences are not met with, regard them as mere exceptions to an all but universal rule. To some extent this opinion has permeated society, and although it has failed in preventing such unions, the popular view has of late years been tending to a conviction that degeneracy of race is to be largely attributed to the union of blood-relations. Thus Duvay, of Lyons, asserts "that in pure consanguinity, isolated from all circumstances of hereditary disease, resides, *ipso facto*, a principle of organic vitiation."

On the other hand, a not inconsiderable section regard this conclusion with doubt, and teach that consanguineous unions may be effected with impunity. We may place, as representing this party, and in antithetical relation to that of Duvay, the assertion of Dr. Gilbert Child, that "the marriages of blood-relations have no tendency, *per se*, to produce degeneration of race."

The arguments of the former are drawn from examples of a somewhat isolated character, and, in the language of their opponents, "attempt often to prove too much." No one, I think, with a previously unbiassed mind, can read the numerous examples which are cited to prove as the result of such unions sterility, deaf-mutism, idiocy, and other characteristics of degeneration, without coming to the conclusion that the cases from which they argue are selected ones, and that the cause they advocate is damaged by special pleading where there should have been judicial deliberation. Writing from a standpoint of observation which enables me to give an opinion on the subject, and having regard to a great deal that has been written, I cannot but join Dr. Child in his very just remark, "to say that all but half the children of the marriages of cousins are idiotic, is simply to say the cases from which the statistics were drawn are not fair cases."

The arguments of the party, of which I have placed Dr. Child as the exponent, are mainly based on observations on the results of the modern system of breeding among the lower animals, and on the examples furnished by the Hebrew race and the North American Indians.

The racial degeneracy, which it is the purpose of this paper to examine in its relation to consanguineous unions, is that congenital mental defect, which, manifesting itself in different varieties as to intensity, has received the name of idiocy.

My notes refer to 1138 cases of idiots, 753 being males, and 385 females, which I may say *en passant* is about the ratio, according to my experience, in which the sexes are affected by idiocy, viz. in the proportion of about two to one.

I have taken the records with every care as to accuracy, and from the number have excluded all cases in which there was impossibility in obtaining information or elements of doubt when obtained. Influenced only by these circumstances, I have eliminated 196 males and 90 females, leaving 557 males and 295 females, or a total of 852, on which the arguments will be based.

Of the 753 male idiots, 33 were the progeny of first cousins; in two of these instances there was another element elicited, viz. in one case the mother was also the product of first cousins, and in the other the mother was the product of cousins germain, involving, therefore, in these two cases, an increased intensity of blood-relationship. Three cases were the progeny of second cousins. Four of third cousins. In all, 40 cases out of 753, or only rather more than 5 per cent., could by any possibility have been due to consanguineous unions. Of the 295 females, 13 were the progeny of first cousins, 3 were the children of second, and 4 those of third cousins. In all, 20 among 295, or little less than 7 per cent., could have been caused by the marriage of blood-relations.

The difference in the percentage of idiots, the progeny of cousins, between the male and female sex is remarkable, but may, I think, be explained by the existence of a preponderating cause of idiocy on the part of males over females, in the larger size of the male cranium at birth, and the consequent greater risk of injury to the cranial contents during parturition.

I am unable to say with certainty how frequently the marriage of blood-relations takes place in an ordinary community, but I have made a careful inquiry into the family history of 200 persons, collected from different districts, who are sane and healthy, and who belong to different families, and I find only one is the offspring of cousins; being half per cent., and I learn that in that one instance he is the son of unusually healthy parents. Certainly, in his case, there is no symptom of either physical or mental degeneracy, and he would probably be selected from among the 200 as one of the most robust and vigorous.

I propose now, further, to inquire into the cases of idiocy from which my statistics are drawn, and endeavour to discover if there are any other factors, besides that of consanguinity, to account for the manifestation. For this purpose I quote from the notes of 20 cases taken, without selection, from my portfolio, and which may, therefore, be fairly regarded as typical of the whole.

Case 1.—J. V. T., male, born in London, father and mother healthy and of sound mind, but first cousins. The father's mother had hemiplegia at 73. Mother was frightened when six weeks advanced in pregnancy by seeing her mother with paralysis, and to this she attributes the idiocy of the son, who is a microcephale. Three sisters, all healthy. J. V. T. is the fourth, and last born.

Case 2.—M. M. Y., female, born at Calne, father and mother first cousins. The mother's parents were also distantly related. The father healthy and of sound mind, but his brothers and sisters with consumptive tendencies. The mother died from tumour of the brain, several of her relatives died from consumption. M. M. Y. is the second-born and a twin, the other twin healthy and of sound mind. This child was remarkably small when born, is deaf, and had fits for many years. She has one cousin who is demented from epilepsy.

Case 3.—A. E. V. S., male, born at Walworth. The father and mother were first cousins. The father was delicate, sound in mind, but intemperate, his relations healthy. The mother healthy and of sound mind, had given birth to twins twice, her family generally consumptive. A. E. V. S. is the eighth-born, and one of his brothers died from consumption. The mother was frightened by a cat during the seventh month of her pregnancy, and was ill a week in consequence. She attributes the idiocy to her husband's habitual intemperance.

Case 4.—M. A. S., female, born in London. Father and mother first cousins. Father of sound mind, died from pulmonary hæmorrhage. One of his sisters died from consumption. Mother consumptive, has also lost one sister from consumption. M. A. S. is the fifth-born, and had four brothers and one sister, all have died from consumption.

CASE 5.—F. H., female, born in Lancashire. Father and mother were second cousins. The father healthy and of sound mind; his father lost his sight when a young man (amaurosis ?), two brothers died from consumption. Mother healthy and of sound mind, her aunt on father's side insane. The mother married twice, the first time to a person not related, and had three children, two girls healthy, and one boy who has epileptic fits. She afterwards married her second cousin and had two girls, who are healthy, then a boy, who is decidedly idiotic, and then F. H., who has little or no mental power. F. H. is the seventh-born. Mother states that she believes the cause of the idiocy of the first idiot child was from fright, and that of the second from thinking of the idiocy of the former.

CASE 6.—C. E. H., female, born in Leicestershire. Father and mother first cousins. Father is a clerk in holy orders, healthy now, but was very delicate when at college; his uncle was imbecile, his father was eccentric, and acquired drinking habits, his aunt died from phthisis. The mother is very deaf, her sister died from

MARRIAGES OF CONSANGUINITY. 193

cancer. C. E. H. has three brothers and two sisters of average physical and mental power. She was the first-born, and during the pregnancy the mother had great anxiety about pecuniary matters. The forceps were employed at parturition, and the head was greatly crushed.

CASE 7.—J. C., female, born in Surrey. Father and mother second cousins. Father had fits when a child, is very ailing, and feeble in mind. No family history. The mother not very strong, lost a brother from consumption. J. C. is the sixth-born; her eldest brother died from acute hydrocephalus; the rest are all bright although not very strong. The mother says she saw, when seven months advanced in pregnancy, a girl precisely like her daughter both mentally and physically.

CASE 8.—J. T. B., male, born at Wingham. Father and mother third cousins; father healthy and of sound mind, very deaf; his cousin became blind from study. Mother healthy, but all her relations consumptive. J. T. B. is the seventh-born, and is a twin-child; his twin-sister is very intelligent, as are also another sister and eight brothers.

CASE 9.—E. P. C., male, born at Tiverton. Father and mother first cousins; father died from Bright's disease after five years' illness; relations healthy. Mother healthy, but nervous; had bad health during her pregnancy, and was much distressed by her eldest child having croup in Paris, and not being able to procure a doctor. She had a very bad labour, owing to the large size of the child. There are two brothers and three sisters, all particularly intelligent. E. P. C. is the fourth-born.

CASE 10.—W. G., male, born at Dorking. Father and mother were second cousins. Father healthy, and of sound mind; has lost five brothers and sisters from consumption, and has one sister insane. The mother has had a fistula, is of sound mind. She was very low-spirited during pregnancy at the prospect of another child, with limited means for the support of the family. W. G. is the fourth-born, and has had three brothers and two sisters; one brother died from scarlatina, one is rather delicate, the rest are healthy and intelligent.

CASE 11.—W. A. P., male, born at Peckham. Father and mother first cousins. The father was healthy, but below the average in mental power; his relations were healthy. The mother has always been delicate, and is very nervous, had an aunt insane, all her brothers and sisters died young. W. A. P. is the eleventh-born, and has had four brothers and six sisters. The first-born, a male, is an idiot, one brother died of inflammation of the lungs, one of convulsions at a fortnight old. Four sisters are dead—two were twins, one died at birth, and the other twin-child, when ten days old, of fits, one died from fever; there are two sisters and one brother living, who are all intelligent.

CASE 12.—W. R., male, born in London. Father and mother were first cousins. Father has good health, but is very irritable and desponding; his mother died of consumption, and he lost one sister from congestion of the brain. Mother healthy, has lost one sister from consumption, and has an uncle imbecile. The mother suffered severely from sea-sickness when in the fourth month of pregnancy. The umbilical cord was obliged to be divided before the birth, animation was suspended and had to be resuscitated by artificial means. W. R. is the eleventh-born, has had eleven brothers and sisters, all of whom had average mental and bodily power.

CASE 13.—R. S., male, born in London. Father and mother first cousins. The father healthy, sober, and steady, family healthy. The mother suffers from chronic bronchitis, sound in mind, and family healthy. The relative ages of father and mother at the birth of R. S. were 41 and 29. The labour was lingering, and ergot of rye given twice; the head was misshapen, and the child made a strange noise when born. R. S. is the fourth-born, and has had one brother and seven sisters. One had no bone on one side of the head, and lived only two days; four died at birth, but seemed all right. The rest quite healthy children. The first three born are the healthy ones, the rest have all been defective or have died. The mother miscarried with a child with one leg.

CASE 14.—J. B., male, born at Tottenham. The father and mother were first cousins. The father has good health, but is of low intelligence; his relations healthy. The mother is delicate, and lost a brother and sister from consumption. J. B. was the third-born, and had one brother and four sisters; one boy had fits and died from consumption, one girl died from epilepsy at seven years, the rest healthy and bright.

CASE 15.—E. P., male, born at Bath. The father and mother are second cousins. The father has average health, but is a drunkard, six of his immediate relatives stammer. The mother has very poor health, and suffers from uterine disease; two of her sisters died young from consumption. The mother was ill during the whole of her pregnancy, fell downstairs during the seventh month, was nervous, and was disturbed by hallucinations. E. P. was the second-born, and had three brothers and three sisters; one died of water on the brain, one of scarlet fever, and one of consumption. Three are idiots.

CASE 16.—J. A. V., male, born in London. Father and mother are first cousins. Father is healthy, but his father was eight months in an asylum with mania, and recovered; father's mother very eccentric; his sister had spinal disease, and died from consumption. Mother healthy, but nearly all her immediate relatives consumptive. She had much trouble and business difficulties during her pregnancy. J. A. V. is the fourth-born, had two brothers and one sister who were intelligent.

Case 17.—J. T. W., male, born in London. Father and mother are first cousins. Father is a very weak and nervous man, faints frequently, and his whole bearing is like one suffering from mercurial tremor. The mother has good health, but is very nervous, her mother is also nervous, and bordering on being insane, one uncle died insane, and one cousin is imbecile. She fell downstairs when six months pregnant, and about the same time she was much frightened by her husband falling down in a fainting fit, which induced in her uterine action and a considerable amount of flooding. J. T. W. is the first-born, and has had five brothers; one died from a fit during an attack of whooping-cough, one died from bronchitis, one is paralysed on one side, and another is three years and a half old, and cannot talk, is only just able to walk, and has a large head.

CASE 18.—E. H. H., male, born at Lewes. Father and mother were first cousins. Father is healthy, but irritable; one of his sisters died from consumption, and another, who also died from consumption, was subject to delusions. The mother died from consumption, and had an uncle who suffered from dementia, thought to have been induced by drink. She was frightened two months before her confinement by stepping on an adder. The labour was lingering, and the child's head much distorted. E. H. H. was the first-born, and was born with animation suspended; he had one sister only, who was prematurely born, and who died three days after her birth.

CASE 19.—G. K., male, born at Woolwich. Father and mother were first cousins. Father is healthy, and of sound mind; his relatives were of average health and mental power. Mother healthy, and of sound mind; her mother was insane; her aunt died in an asylum; and another aunt's child suffers after every confinement from puerperal mania. G. K. was the second-born, and had one brother and three sisters; one sister is an idiot, and another was quite helpless, and died at the age of fourteen months.

CASE 20.—T. R., male, born at Thetford, Norfolk. Father and mother were first cousins. Father died from a contraction of the bowel, sound in mind, and steady; his mother used to stammer; mother very nervous; she was frightened during her pregnancy by seeing an idiotic man. Labour lasted twenty-eight hours, and she was delivered with instruments. T. R. is the first-born, and had three brothers and one sister; one brother died from whooping-cough; the second and third were twins, and are very healthy; all sound in mind.

My own statistics differ so much from those published by Dr. Howe, of the United States, and on which many arguments have been based, that I am induced to place them in contrast:—

Dr. Howe's 17 marriages produced 95 children—*i.e.* 5·58 each. Of the 95 children—

MARRIAGES OF CONSANGUINITY.

37 were of tolerable health.
1 was a dwarf.
1 was deaf.
12 were scrofulous or puny.
44 were idiots.

Total 95

Thus more than 46 per cent. were idiots.

'The 20 marriages, relating to my own cases, produced 138 children—*i. e.* 6·9 each. Of the 138 children—

75 had average health and intellect.
11 were consumptive.
8 were still-born.
4 died from convulsions or fits.
2 were hydrocephalic.
7 died young from infantile complaints.
6 were puny and delicate.
25 were idiots.

Total 138

It will be seen that only a little more than 18 per cent. were idiots.

It will be interesting to place also in contrast the results of 20 marriages, in which there was no consanguinity, but in which there were one or more instances of mental defect in the progeny of each family, and which have been taken, like the former twenty cases, from a much larger number, without any principle of selection. The 20 non-sanguineous marriages produced 145 children, or 7·25 each. Of the 145 children—

    83 had average health.
    1 was consumptive.
    11 were still-born.
    3 died from convulsions or fits.
    2 were hydrocephalic.
    13 died from infantile complaints.
    6 were puny, or dwarfed.
    26 were idiots.

Total 145

It will be seen that 18 per cent. were idiots. In the case of the consanguineous progeny, 55 per cent. were of average health; in the non-consanguineous, 57 per cent. No one, I think, who has had an opportunity of investigating the subject, or who compares these statistics with Dr. Howe's, can avoid coming to the conclusion that Dr. Howe's 17 cases were not typical of what is to be met with in this country. Only 39 per cent. of the progeny in his cases had average health.

I have shown that about 6 per cent. of those suffering from congenital mental defect are the product of consanguineous marriages, while, among the healthy and vigorous, only about half per cent. may be placed as the result of such unions. One cannot, therefore, resist the conviction that the union of blood-relations has some influence in the deterioration of our species. What that influence is, however, can only be determined by a further investigation into the etiology of the 20 cases I have cited.

Out of the 20 cases, among whom the average number of children were 6·9 each, no less than 5, or 25 per cent., were primiparæ. This of itself, according to my observation, is sometimes a cause of idiocy. It may be explained, I believe, by the greater injury sustained in the birth than at subsequent labours, and is analogous to the determining cause of the preponderance of male over female idiots before alluded to.* No less important is the fact,

* In the statistics of the maternity department of the London Hospital ('London Hospital Reports,' vol. i,

that in two cases the forceps were employed at the birth of the child, or in 10 per cent. of the cases. I find from the statistical report of the maternity department of the London Hospital, by Mr. Heckford, published in the first volume of the 'London Hospital Reports,' that the forceps were employed only in 8 per cent. of the children alive. It would not be difficult to prove, by reference to all the notes I possess, that instrumental interference is of itself a cause of idiocy. In two of the 20 cases, in which instruments were not employed, the head of the child was much missphapen by the difficulty of the labour.

One was a twin-child, and there is reason to believe that this condition may, of itself, be conducive to defective mental development. Suspended animation was reported in two cases, or 10 per cent.; how far this may influence the future development of the child, I shall inquire into, in a future paper.

Ergot of rye was given in one case; but I am not aware of any observations on the use of this drug as a cause of idiocy.

p. 254), it is stated that the stillborn males exceeded the females by 35 per cent.

This disposes of all the possible causes influencing the child at parturition. I have now to inquire into the hereditary influences which might have affected the ovum, and I think it will be readily granted that no breeder of cattle, apart from all question of breeding in and in, would select analogous stock for propagation from, to those which constitute the parents of the twenty cases I have quoted.

Thus, among the progenitors of the twenty, in no fewer than twelve instances, was phthisis abundantly established in the family history of one or both parents.

In 12 cases there was well-established history of insanity, epilepsy, or imbecility in the family of one or both progenitors reaching to the large amount of 60 per cent. In 2 cases the fathers were habitual drunkards. In one instance the mother was very deaf, and the same case furnished the solitary example of cancer.

There were only 4 cases in which there did not exist either a history of insanity or phthisis in the family. In the first of these the father's mother stammered when young, the mother stated that she was nervous during her pregnancy, during which she was frightened by an idiotic man. The boy had four brothers and sisters, all of whom were healthy, and he was one of the cases delivered by forceps. In the second case there was no history of hereditary taint. There was, however, disparity in the ages of the parents: father was 41 and the mother 29. The labour was very lingering, and it was the one case in which ergot of rye was administered.*

In the third case, the father was suffering from Bright's disease at the time of procreation, from which disease he died.

The fourth case is the only one in which the consanguinity stands as an isolated cause, and even in this instance there are three sisters perfectly sound, and it is the only example of degeneracy in the family, while the mother asserts that she was frightened by seeing her mother with paralysis at the age of 73. It is worthy of remark that the father's mother also died from paralysis at the age of 70. The boy is a microcephale and the last-born; the father, about the time of the procreation, grew thrift-

---

* Dr. Ramsbotham has shown that the ergot of rye influences unfavorably the viability of the child.

less, ran away to Australia, and has not been heard of.

It is also noteworthy that these four exceptional examples are all males. Reviewing the whole of these cases, there is only one, and that the one just mentioned, in which there is not quite sufficient to account for the idiocy apart from consanguineous influences.

Since writing the foregoing, my attention has been called to a paper of Dr. Mitchell's, read before the Medico-Chirurgical Society of Edinburgh,* in which, making observations from a similar point of view to myself, on a different field, he has arrived at very opposite conclusions. He found in Scotland that more than every sixth idiot born in wedlock was the child of cousins. I am unable to account for such a wide disparity, and in the face of it can only reiterate the care with which my information has been collected, and the impartiality with which my results are here presented. My own researches conclusively show that in England, at least, every fourteenth idiot only is the child of cousins. But can it be as certainly

* 'Edin. Med. Journ.,' vol. viii, p. 872.

shown that the relationship *per se* is the cause of the idiocy? I think not, and the analysis I have made clearly shows that in the vast majority of such, so great in fact that it may almost be said to be universal, other causes were operating which were merely intensified by the relationship. Had the same care been exercised in the selection of relations as is displayed by the breeder of race-horses, vastly different results might have ensued; or were the practice of the coloured races of North America in force, of destroying all the weak, rachitic, and diseased children, the intermarriage of cousins would not have displayed the facts which I have furnished. Consanguinity has doubtless the power of aggravating any morbid tendency, as I believe it has of perfecting any good quality. Any statistics on the results of the marriage of relations are of doubtful value unless they give the life-history of the progenitors. What a different aspect the whole matter assumes when this plan is adopted, will be apparent to the readers of this paper. Whenever a similar investigation is made, I believe it will be found, as in the subjects of my own inquiry, that consanguinity is only *one* of the factors, and not the most important one, in the production of deterioration.

If our advice is sought, it will be our duty to inquire into other elements which are less on the surface, but which have equal or even greater potentiality for evil.

Alliances, such as I have exhibited, with hereditary disease on both sides, should be discountenanced even where there is no element of consanguinity. It would only be a part of a true philosophy to render more forcible our opposition where blood-relationship would have a well-determined tendency to aggravate the wrong.

OBSERVATIONS

ON AN

ETHNIC CLASSIFICATION OF IDIOTS.

'London Hospital Reports,' 1866.

THOSE who have given any attention to congenital mental lesions must have been frequently puzzled how to arrange, in any satisfactory way, the different classes of this defect which have come under their observation. Nor will the difficulty be lessened by an appeal to what has been written on the subject. The systems of classification are generally so vague and artificial that not only do they assist but feebly in any mental arrangement of the phenomena which are presented, but they completely fail in exerting any practical influence on the subject.

The medical practitioner who may be consulted in any given case, has, perhaps in a very early condition of the child's life, to give an opinion on points of vital importance as to the present condition and probable future of the little one. Moreover, he may be pressed as to the question, whether the supposed defect dates from any cause subsequent to the birth or not. Has the nurse dosed the child with opium? Has the little one met with any accident? Has the instrumental interference which maternal safety demanded been the cause of what seems to the anxious parents a vacant future? Can it be that when away from the family attendant medicine has been injudiciously prescribed? Can, in fact, the strange anomalies which the child presents be attributed to the numerous causes which maternal solicitude conjures to the imagination, in order to account for a condition, for which *any* cause is sought rather than hereditary taint or parental influence? Will the systems of classification, either all together, or any one of them, assist the medical adviser in the opinion he is to present, or the suggestions which he is to tender to the anxious parent? I think that they will entirely fail him in the matter, and that he will have in many cases to make a *guarded* diagnosis and prognosis, so guarded, in fact as to be almost valueless; or to venture an authoritative assertion which the future may or may not confirm.

I have for some time had my attention directed to the possibility of making a classification of the feeble-minded, by arranging them around various ethnic standards,—in other words, framing a natural system to supplement the information to be derived by an inquiry into the history of the case.

I have been able to find among the large number of idiots and imbeciles which come under my observation, both at Earlswood and the out-patient department of the hospital, that a considerable portion can be fairly referred to one of the great divisions of the human family other than the class from which they have sprung. Of course there are numerous representatives of the great Caucasian family. Several well-marked examples of the Ethiopian variety have come under my notice, presenting the characteristic malar bones, the prominent eyes, the puffy lips, and retreating chin. The woolly hair has also been present, although not

CLASSIFICATION OF IDIOTS. 213

always black, nor has the skin acquired pigmentary deposit. They have been specimens of white negroes, although of European descent.

Some arrange themselves around the Malay variety, and present in their soft, black, curly hair, their prominent upper jaws and capacious mouths, types of the family which people the South Sea Islands.

Nor have there been wanting the analogues of the people who, with shortened foreheads, prominent cheeks, deep-set eyes, and slightly apish nose, originally inhabited the American Continent.

The great Mongolian family has numerous representatives, and it is to this division I wish, in this paper, to call special attention. A very large number of congenital idiots are typical Mongols. So marked is this that, when placed side by side, it is difficult to believe that the specimens compared are not children of the same parents. The number of idiots who arrange themselves around the Mongolian type is so great, and they present such a close resemblance to one another in mental power, that I shall describe an idiot member of this racial division, selected from the large number that have fallen under my observation.

The hair is not black, as in the real Mongol, but of a brownish colour, straight and scanty. The face is flat and broad, and destitute of prominence. The cheeks are roundish, and extended laterally. The eyes are obliquely placed, and the internal canthi more than normally distant from one another. The palpebral fissure is very narrow. The forehead is wrinkled transversely from the constant assistance which the levatores palpebrarum derive from the occipito-frontalis muscle in the opening of the eyes. The lips are large and thick with transverse fissures. The tongue is long, thick, and much roughened. The nose is small. The skin has a slight dirty yellowish tinge, and is deficient in elasticity, giving the appearance of being too large for the body.

The boy's aspect is such that it is difficult to realise that he is the child of Europeans, but so frequently are these characters presented that there can be no doubt that these ethnic features are the result of degeneration.

The Mongolian type of idiocy occurs in more than 10 per cent. of the cases which are presented to me. They are always congenital idiots, and never result from accidents after uterine life. They are, for the most part, instances of degeneracy arising from tuberculosis in the parents. They are cases which very much repay judicious treatment. They require highly azotised food with a considerable amount of oleaginous material. They have considerable power of imitation, even bordering on being mimics. They are humorous, and a lively sense of the ridiculous often colours their mimicry. This faculty of imitation may be cultivated to a very great extent, and a practical direction given to the results obtained. They are usually able to speak; the speech is thick and indistinct, but may be improved very greatly by a well-directed scheme of tongue gymnastics. The co-ordinating faculty is abnormal, but not so defective that it cannot be greatly strengthened. By systematic training, considerable manipulative power may be obtained.

The circulation is feeble, and however much advance is made intellectually in the summer, some amount of retrogression may be expected in the winter. Their mental and physical capabilities are, in fact, *directly* as the temperature.

The improvement which training effects in them is greatly in excess of what would be predicated if one did not know the characteristics of the type. The life expectancy, however, is far below the average, and the tendency is to the tuberculosis which I believe to be the hereditary origin of the degeneracy.

Apart from the practical bearing of this attempt at an ethnic classification, considerable philosophical interest attaches to it. The tendency in the present day is to reject the opinion that the various races are merely varieties of the human family having a common origin, and to insist that climatic, or other influences, are insufficient to account for the different types of man. Here, however, we have examples of retrogression, or, at all events, of departure from one type and the assumption of the characteristics of another. If these great racial divisions are fixed and definite, how comes it that disease is able to break down the barrier, and to simulate so closely the features of the members of another division? I cannot but think that the observations which I have recorded are indications that the differences in the races are not specific but variable.

These examples of the result of degeneracy among mankind, appear to me to furnish some arguments in favour of the unity of the human species.

ON IDIOCY AND ITS RELATION TO TUBERCULOSIS.

'The Lancet,' vol. ii, 1867.

THE causes which have been assigned as productive of idiocy are numerous, and some have received special advocacy. Thus we are asked to believe that one of the most profound misfortunes which afflicts our race—which to a great extent blots out the characteristics of man, and approximates him to the lower animals —arises from sucking the thumb; and that if we could prevent a "fruitless sucking" idiocy would be immensely diminished, even if it did not cease to exist. Others, with more show of reason, urge the intermarriage of blood relations as the prevailing cause; and so far does a belief in the potency of this latter element permeate society that I have been often gravely asked whether intermarriage of relations is not the cause of the idiocy of three fourths of the cases which come under my observation. No one who has had an opportunity of investigating the influences which are at work in the production of congenital mental diseases can fail to be struck with the fact that they are, for the most part, to be traced to some inherent vice of constitution in the progenitors. He will discover in the parents elements of degeneracy which must have had their share in producing the catastrophe. He will notice how by degrees the stock has deteriorated. He will be able to estimate how intemperance or sensuality leads slowly but surely to idiocy—how physical weakness of the parents culminates in the mental blight of the child.

Amongst the influences which have been regarded as connected with idiocy, very little attention has been given to that of tuberculosis, and I am not aware that any observations have been made with reference to the connection of these two maladies.

Several writers have discussed the relations between insanity and tuberculosis, and have, I think, made it tolerably evident that there is more than an accidental connexion between them.

At the Earlswood Asylum, where the following observations have been made, the subjects of the inquiry are not likely to present an unfair proportion of tubercular idiots. Rather would they be likely to be below the average. The inmates are, for the most part, elected after great exertion, and the friends of a phthisical idiot would scarcely be likely to undertake the trouble for a manifestly short-lived child, even if the rules of the institution did not exclude it.

During the past eight years, from 1859 to 1866 inclusive, there have been 201 deaths. During this time there have been two epidemics of measles, one of scarlet fever, and two of whooping-cough, which have all added to the mortality. Moreover, a large proportion of the patients who succumbed to these epidemic diseases were those who would in all probability have eventually died of phthisis but for their intervention. Notwithstanding this circumstance there remains the fact, which my notes record, that, of the whole mortality, 39·8 is due to phthisis. To appreciate fully the meaning of these figures, it is necessary to consider the rate of mortality which rules amongst an idiot population. My notes show that, taking the last eight years, in some of which there were epidemics, while others were entirely free therefrom, the mortality presented an average of about 73·3 per 1000; whereas the mortality of the district in which the asylum is situated was about 18 per 1000.

Date.	Average population.	Gross mortality.	Deaths from phthisis.	—
1859	285¾	13	7	
1860	308¾	22	7	Epidemic of typhoid.
1861	318⅓	23	13	
1862	322	33	8	Epidemic of measles.
1863	344½	47	15	Epidemic of measles and scarlatina.
1864	369⅚	19	10	
1865	412¾	13	9	
1866	423½	31	11	Epidemic of measles.

The statistics of London show that the deaths from phthisis constitute 115 per 1000 of the general mortality. My notes of the causes of death at Earlswood indicate that phthisis was the actual cause of death in 398 per 1000 of the general mortality. The significance, however, of this, as before observed, can only be rightly estimated by recollecting that the general mortality is four times that of an ordinary community.

It will be obvious that, in consequence of the greater readiness with which idiots succumb to epidemic or other diseases, the proportional deaths from phthisis are thereby much decreased. This element may be fully brought out by dividing the eight years; bringing together the four epidemic years, and comparing them with the four non-epidemic years. It will then be seen that during the epidemic years 1860, 1862, 1863, and 1866, the deaths from phthisis numbered 297 per 1000 of the general mortality, or considerably more than twice the ratio which rules in London; while in the non-epidemic years 1859, 1861, 1864, and 1865, the deaths from phthisis reached the enormous proportion of 570·58 per thousand of the general mortality. I now propose to present a tabular view of the age and sex of those who died from phthisis.

Age.	Male.	Female.	Total.
7	1	0	1
8	1	0	1
9	1	2	3
10	3	0	3

Age.	Male.	Female.	Total.
11	2	1	3
12	3	1	4
13	6	2	8
14	5	2	7
15	1	0	1
16	4	1	5
17	2	6	8
18	4	3	7
19	8	1	9
20	7	1	8
21	6	2	8
23	2	0	2
27	1	0	1
29	1	0	1
	58	22	80

Dividing the ages into quinquennial periods, it will be observed that the greatest mortality from phthisis was from fifteen to twenty years of age.

From 5 to 10 years	8
,, 10 to 15 ,,	23
,, 15 to 20 ,,	38
,, 20 to 25 ,,	10
,, 25 to 30 ,,	2

The above details have reference solely to ante-mortem diagnosis and have included cases where the death was evidently caused by phthisis. I have, however, made an analysis of the last hundred of my post-mortem records, and I find that no fewer than 62 per cent. were subjects of tubercular deposit. There were 62 males, and tubercular deposit was found in 49 instances, or 79·03 per cent. There were 38 females, and of these 13, or 34 per cent., were tubercular.

Dr. Clouston, in the 'Journal of Mental Science' for 1863, has analysed the post-mortem records of the insane at the Royal Edinburgh Asylum, and found that 60·9 per cent. had tubercular deposit. It would appear that idiots are slightly more liable to tuberculosis than the insane, but there is a remarkable difference between the proclivity of the two sexes. While among the insane, 51·7 per cent. of the males were tubercular, 73 per cent. of the females had tubercular deposit. Among idiots, however, while the females have a remarkable immunity, the deposit being found in only 34 per cent., among the males no less than 79·03 per cent., or more than twice the ratio, had tubercle in some of their organs.

If we inquire into the sex of those whose death resulted from phthisis, and in whom the diagnosis was made during life, we shall also find that the females suffered in a less degree than the males. While 31·9 per cent. of the female mortality resulted from phthisis, this disease was the cause of death in 44·6 per cent. of the males.

The following table will give the distribution of the deposit in the different organs :—

Total number of cases referred to, 100.

	Males.	Females.	Total.
Total number of cases found tubercular	37	25	62
Lungs	31	21	52
Lungs, much deposit	24	14	38
Lungs, slight deposit	7	7	14
Deposit in right lung	26	17	43
Deposit in left lung	27	21	48
Peritoneum	4	3	7
Nervous centres	3	3	6
Bronchial glands	12	6	18
Liver	5	4	9
Kidneys	4	0	4
Spleen	7	2	9

It is worthy of remark that tubercle is rarely found in the encephalon. In only two cases did this occur; in one the corpus striatum was the seat of the deposit, and in the other the cerebellum. The most noticeable character observed was the extreme pallor of the cortical substance of the encephalon; and so frequent was this that it was all but universal. Occasional softening of the fornix and the neighbouring parts was met with, but not nearly so frequently as paleness of what should be the grey portion of the brain.

In several of the cases included in the above record, most careful inquiry failed to discover any family history of tuberculosis; and the brothers and sisters were thoroughly vigorous. In these cases the tuberculosis appears to have been the sequence of the idiocy—a condition of idiocy resulting from accidental causes. Defective innervation in all probability led to malnutrition, and predisposed to a tubercular condition. In some this was doubtless materially assisted by the imperfect mastication and insalivation to which the food was subjected. The tendency to bolt the food unmixed with saliva often prevents the proper alteration of the starchy element, so as to fit it for speedy assimilation.

On the other hand, in a large number of cases the progenitors had also manifested a tubercular condition; and in some the tuberculosis of the parents had been, in my opinion, the prime cause of the idiocy of the offspring. I have elsewhere shown ('Lond. Hosp. Reports,' vol. iii) that a specific phase of idiocy—a phase which is curiously associated with altered racial characters—arises from tuberculosis of the progenitors.

The subjects of this class assume the Mongolian type; and while they present a marked similarity in external conformation, they are characterised by the same mental and moral peculiarities; so that, given a case of the Mongolian type, we are often able to trace its origin to tuberculosis, and to predicate the extent of response to training that may be expected, and the tendencies it will evince. Moreover, the knowledge that is gained by this racial character assists in laying down specific rules as to food, medicine, and general hygiene, without which the mental development would be but small. The power of progress is usually much greater than one would judge by an ordinary inspection. Such cases are extremely susceptible to climatic changes, and winter is for them a period of mental and physical developmental rest. In the spring they put forward increased imitative and receptive powers, which compensate to some extent for the period of hybernation.

It will be interesting now to ascertain to what extent tuberculosis exists among the progenitors of idiot children generally. I have gone through my records very carefully, disregarding all doubtful cases, meaning thereby cases in which, although there has been a death from phthisis in the family, I had reason to believe that it arose from accidental causes, and selecting only those in which the tubercular taint was well impressed. I find that in 31 per cent. of the cases of idiocy which have come under my care, or about whom I have been consulted, tuberculosis existed in an unmistakeable manner, in the family of the progenitors; in 6 per cent. the tubercular element was found on both sides of the family; in 10 per cent. it was due to the father; while in 15 per cent. the tuberculosis belonged to the mother. It is a somewhat singular circumstance that while tuberculosis is more frequent on the maternal side, the male progeny are the most tubercular.

In the third volume of the 'London Hospital

Reports,' I have endeavoured to show that idiocy has been too often traced to the intermarriage of blood relations, without regarding other elements that may be operative. It is readily conceivable that if there be tuberculosis strongly impressed on a family, the members of that family would by intermarriage be taking tolerably effectual steps to ensure the extinction of their race. Certain it is that in a large number of the cases in which marriages of consanguinity are referred to as the cause of idiocy, the tuberculosis of the progenitors is a potent, but often disregarded, element. The Mongolian type, which I have elsewhere described, occurs, according to my observation, in greater degree when the tubercular element is strongly impressed, still more where it exists in both branches of the family, and greatest if consanguinity is added thereto.

It appears to me that tuberculosis must be accepted as one important cause of idiocy ; that it impresses special characters thereon, characters which impart a strong family likeness to the subjects of this class.

It is no less clear to me that idiocy of a non-tubercular origin leads to tuberculosis. Whether this arises through the influence of the pneumogastric nerve, mal-assimilation of food, or defective innervation, it cannot but be regarded that the connection between these two maladies is by no means accidental, and that a due appreciation of this relation is necessary to those who would treat effectively congenital mental lesions.

A CASE

OF

ASYMMETRICALLY DEVELOPED BRAIN.

'Trans. Path. Soc.,' 1869.

THE brain now exhibited was removed from the cranium of a girl seventeen years of age, who had been idiotic from birth. Her father died insane. Her mother had good bodily and mental health. She was the youngest of six children. The other members of the family had average intellectual powers, but were all delicate as to their physical health; one brother died from phthisis. At the age of seven months she had epileptic fits, which persisted for some time at short intervals. She never spoke. The cutting of her teeth and her walking were both deferred. She was passionate and self-willed. She was always in motion, full of mischief, and delighted in tearing things up and putting them on the fire. Her habits were dirty. Under the influence of training she became clean, tractable, and able to take some part in her own toilet. She was taught to feed herself with propriety at table. She made no attempt to speak, apparently from want of ideas to communicate. She would come when called, but manifested very little affection. Her demeanour indicated considerable erotic feeling. There was no paralysis either of sensation or motion, and her powers of prehension and manipulation were susceptible of education.

Her physical health had been very good for several years, until an attack of scarlet fever led to acute desquamative nephritis, and consequent broncho-pneumonia.

Post-mortem examination.—The body was well nourished, and weighed 6 stones 12 lbs. There was hair on the pubis, but not in the axillæ. The heart weighed $7\frac{1}{2}$ oz., the valves competent; the large vessels filled with clots of blood. The left lung was adherent to the costal pleura, weighing $14\frac{3}{4}$ oz.; interlobular adhesions. The apex was much puckered, corresponding thereto was a calcareous mass the size of a pea, of a hard density; another part of the apex contained a tubercular nodule the size of a bean. The posterior part of the lung was intensely congested. The right lung was hepatised throughout $\frac{7}{8}$ of its extent. The bronchial glands were enlarged, and the tubes intensely injected. The kidneys presented at the margin of the pyramids a deep red colour. The uterus and ovaries were normal.

The cranium was slightly unsymmetrical, exhibiting slight flattening on the anterior third of the left side. The circumference was $21\frac{3}{4}$ in.; the antero-posterior diameter 6·5 in.; the antero-posterior curve $10\frac{3}{4}$ in.; the bilateral diameter 5·3 in.; the bilateral curve 7·5 in. On removing the calvarium the anterior portion of the left side corresponding to the external flattening was found to be enormously thickened.

The left side of the encephalon was consequently much smaller than the right, and on removing the brain it was found that this disparity was still further increased by a diminution of brain matter on the inferior surface of the anterior lobe, which was replaced by excessive thickening and consequent elevation of the orbital plate of the frontal bone.

The left hemisphere was not more than two-thirds the size of the right. The occipital lobe was slightly less developed on the left side than on the right, but the great cause of want of symmetry was the absence of development of the frontal lobe. All the convolutions were present, but the middle and inferior frontal gyri were extremely minute in size, although not more simple than usual. The gyri of the orbital lobule were also of small size.

Remarks.—Asymmetrical brains are not unfrequently met with in dissections of idiots, but so great an inequality has never before come under my notice. There was no want of symmetry in the lobes of the cerebellum. In this case it was arrest of growth rather than of development, as indicated by the complexity of the defective convolutions. The amount of disparity could not have been predicated before death by external examination of the cranium. The thickened calvarium and orbital plate were sequential to and not antecedent to the arrested growth.

A remarkable case of asymmetrical brain, which came under my notice a few years since, had associated with it an asymmetrical cranium, but the larger side of cranium corresponded to the diminished hemisphere of the encephalon; the inner and outer tables of the skull had separated widely, so that external examination gave no idea of the size of the skull cavity.

It is worthy of remark that the region implicated was that known as Broca's. Having regard, however, to the frequency of absence of speech in idiocy, I cannot look upon this case as being of much importance in localising the faculty of speech to one half of the hemisphere, or to the frontal lobe in particular. The absence of speech was the result of defect of cerebration generally. There was no power to formulate ideas, and speech was not required. It should also be noticed that she was the *youngest* child of a father who died insane. There is reason to believe that she was procreated during the early progress of the mental alienation, and thus suffered in a way different from the others, who were born anterior to the mental change. This is in accordance with many instances which have come under my observation, and what might be theoretically expected.

A CASE

OF

MICROCEPHALIC SKULL.

'Trans. Path. Soc.,' 1869.

THE cranium exhibited is that of a boy thirteen years of age, having a height of 45½ inches, and a weight of 26 lbs., who died from tubercular disease of the lungs. He was the son of healthy parents, but had been an idiot from birth. The cause of idiocy was attributed to fright of the mother during pregnancy. He was dirty in his habits, did not speak, and was extremely mischievous. The circumference of his head measured 18 inches, the longitudinal curve 11 inches, the longitudinal diameter 6 inches, the bilateral curve 10 inches, the bilateral diameter 4·8 inches; the brain weighed 2½ lbs.; the fornix was diffluent, the middle commissure absent, the right corpus striatum smaller than the left; the pons Varolii and medulla oblongata weighed together $\frac{3}{4}$ oz.; the cerebellum weighed $3\frac{3}{4}$ oz., the right lobe being narrower anteriorly than the left. The calvarium, when deprived of integument, measured 17 inches; the longitudinal diameter $5\frac{7}{8}$ inches, the bilateral diameter $4\frac{6}{8}$ inches. The calvarium was unsymmetrical, being larger on the left side posteriorly, and the left parietal eminence being more prominent than the right. The anterior portion of the cranium had a remarkable prow-shaped prominence, corresponding to the medio-frontal suture which remained unossified; all the remaining sutures were in the same condition.

Remarks.—The above case is interesting, not as exhibiting a very extreme degree of microcephalism, but as evidence that premature synostosis of the cranial sutures cannot be regarded as the cause of the abnormal condition. In this case, not only were the usual sutures in an unossified condition; but the medio-frontal suture, which usually becomes ossified during the first year of extra-uterine life, was patent, so that deferred rather than premature synostosis existed. Moreover, it throws doubt on the view usually entertained, that scaphocephalic skulls depend on the premature ossification of the sagittal suture, as in this case the marked frontal ridge corresponded to a line where synostosis had been remarkably postponed.

A CASE

OF

MICROCEPHALIC SKULL.

'Trans. Path. Soc.,' 1869.

The cause of deformation of the cranium, and especially of that kind known as microcephalism, has been so authoritatively stated to be premature synostosis of the cranial sutures, that the tendency has been to acquiesce in this explanation and to accept this as the great determining factor. My own observations on the crania of about 200 idiots—many of them deformed in various ways, and some of them unusually small—have led me to take an entirely different view, and to assume that the deviations of the cranium have been rather the sequence of circumstances arresting the development and growth of the encephalon, and have not been the result of premature ossification of the sutures. The only case in which I have met with ossification of the sutures was a case of macrocephalism, where certainly the ossification of the sutures could have had no influence in the production of the enlarged cephalic mass.

The cranium which I now produce is interesting, as showing how an extreme degree of microcephalism can exist without any ossification of the cranial sutures. The cranium is that of a male, eighteen years of age, who had been educated with some slight result. He had acquired speech and correct habits, had learned to be self-helpful, to count, and to make imitative drawings of a simple character on a black-board. The head measured in its circumference 15 inches. The antero-posterior curve measured from the glabella of the frontal bone over the vertex to the occipital protuberance 8 inches. The bilateral curve over the vertex from above the implantation of the ears was 8 inches. The antero-posterior diameter of the head was 5 inches, the bilateral diameter 3·9 inches.

The greatest antero-posterior diameter of the interior of the cranium was 4·7 inches; the greatest bilateral diameter of the interior of the cranium 3·4 inches.

All the sutures which are usually unossified were perfectly free from synostoses, and, in fact, the cranial bones were more than usually freely separable the one from the other.

It is worthy of remark that more than one foreign observer had predicated during the youth's life that it was a good illustration of premature synostosis. I had been led to doubt this from the result of former autopsies, and I am desirous of placing on record this extreme degree of microcephalism, without any synostosis, as a striking example in which other than mere mechanical causes must be looked for as productive of this and analogous cases.

A CASE

OF

ARRESTED DEVELOPMENT.

'Trans. Path. Soc.,' 1869.

J. P., a female, aged five, came under my observation at the London Hospital. She measured twenty-two inches in height, was unable to walk, but could stand by the help of a chair. She could not speak, and gave utterance only to a few monosyllabic sounds. There was no deformity of the body or limbs. The face had an earthy complexion, and the integument generally had a wrinkled appearance as if it were too large for the diminutive body. The hair was sparse and coarse, the eyebrows obliquely placed, the tongue large and rugous. There was a small tumour on each side of the neck above the clavicle. She understood what was said to her, and had the mental condition of a child about fifteen months old. The father and mother had been healthy, and there was no history of mental or physical deviation on either side. The mother stated that her first child was perfectly healthy, until it died from measles. The husband about that time gave himself up to intemperance, and the mother subsequently gave birth to a child, which died at the age of three, having the same physical peculiarities as the subject of these remarks. The third child, now under consideration, was procreated like the second, while the husband was suffering from alcoholic intoxication. A miscarriage succeeded. The husband at this time relinquished his habits of intemperance, became as thrifty and prudent as he was formerly the reverse; and the wife again becoming pregnant, gave birth to a child normally developed, and in good bodily and mental health, now sixteen months old.

Remarks.—The above case is of great interest, because, in the author's opinion, it adds another to a group of cases which have come under his observation of arrested development arising from intoxication of one or both of the progenitors at the time of the procreative act. The whole group of cases has presented features of such close resemblance that it is difficult to avoid the conclusion that there was some unity of cause, and careful investigation has elicited facts bearing on the etiology of these cases, having a close parallelism to the circumstances, which he believes to have been potential in this. He has known some of these cases to attain the age of twenty, while still preserving infantile characteristics.

In each case the tumours in the neck have been observed.

A CASE OF PARALYSIS

WITH

APPARENT MUSCULAR HYPERTROPHY.

'Path. Soc. Trans.,' 1870.

BENJAMIN ROUND, aged eleven, admitted into the London Hospital, September 14th, 1869.

History.—His mother states that this disorder has been coming on for five years. The first thing wrong which she noticed was, that when he fell down he could not get up again. About two years ago he began to get unsteady in his gait; when running, if he tried to stop himself suddenly, he fell down, and even when walking he had difficulty in stopping without tumbling over. Running was easier to him than walking, and walking than standing still. When he stood still, he looked out for something to lean against, getting to the wall if he could. His mother noticed that as he ran he used to stick out his belly and throw back his shoulders. For the past twelve months he has been unable to walk, and for the past seven months has been gradually losing the use of his arms.

Family history.—His mother's health has always been good, and so has his father's. No history of any hereditary disease, except that his grandfather died from " consumption," and his father's grandfather was insane. All his brothers and sisters are healthy.

The only previous illness the boy has had was measles seven years ago. Has never had thrush nor any cutaneous eruption. Has had thread-worms for six years. His mother suckled him for eighteen months. He was not any longer teething or learning to walk than the other children. He has always been very fat; his belly has always been big, and the calves of his legs have always been large. During the last four years his mother thinks his ankles and thighs have wasted. His head is unusually large. During the past two years he has not been well fed; the family have only had meat once a week, and then a pound and a half divided among ten.

Present condition.—He is utterly unable to

stand. When put upon his legs they sprawl helplessly in every direction. He can sit up, but if he is gently pushed back he falls quite passively upon the floor, and can by no efforts raise himself. As he sits up, he likes to support himself by using his hands as props. When pushed back in bed against the pillow, so that he does not fall quite down, he can manage to raise himself by swinging his head laterally to the front. There is great loss of power over the arms. On being desired to raise his arm slowly, he can move it but a little distance from his side, and that by the aid of his scapular muscles, the shoulder being raised and thrown forward, and the lower angle of the scapula tilted upwards and outwards. By a jerk he can raise it about 60 degrees, and by swinging his arm backwards and forwards, he can get it up nearly horizontally. If his arm be extended in the supine position he can flex it at the elbow-joint, but if a small book be placed in his hand he cannot raise it. If his arm be flexed at the elbow he can extend it, but a weight of three or four ounces prevents his doing so. He can perform any movements with his fingers and thumb, but without much power. When he wishes to raise his hand he does so by the aid of his fingers, making them climb, as it were, over his body and head, and drag his arm after them. He separates his fingers, and places his thumb on a higher point than the rest; he then approximates his fingers, and resting his little finger on the same level as his thumb, again separates his fingers, and plants his thumb on a higher level still; in this way he makes his arm travel to the desired place. He cannot flex the thigh upon the trunk at all in bed; out of bed he can do it a little. As he lies in bed he moves his lower extremities about by the movements of his feet, alternately using the heel and toe as a fixed point to advance the rest of the foot. He can rotate the limb at the hip-joint. Out of bed, by swinging his legs, he can get them to an angle of about forty-five degrees from the perpendicular, but he cannot keep them in opposition to the force of gravity. He can also swing his feet laterally. He can move his feet a little laterally at the ankle-joint, but without much power. He flexes and extends his toes readily. He can adduct the limb slightly, but appears to do so by the action of his quadriceps.

Muscular system; lower extremities. — The

muscles supplied by the gluteal and great sciatic nerves are immensely hypertrophied. On looking at the boy the prominence of his gluteal region is very apparent, and on feeling the part the extreme hardness of the muscle is very striking. The lumbo-sacral curve is greatly exaggerated. The tensor vaginæ femoris can be felt as a thick, hard, firm band under the skin. The flexors of the thighs are also much hypertrophied. The muscles of the calves are also very hard and very large. The extensor and peronei muscles on the outside of the tibia appear to share this hypertrophy. The foot is in a state of talipes equino-varus.

The adductor muscles on the inside of the thigh are very soft, small, and lax. The quadriceps extensor appears somewhat hypertrophied, but it is very difficult to estimate its size. The sartorius is wasted.

Measurements of lower extremities—
    From one iliac spine to the other .= 8 in.
    Around pelvis, over most prominent
        part of glutæi . . . .= $24\frac{1}{2}$ in.
    From anterior superior iliac spine
        to outer condyle. . . .= $12\frac{1}{4}$ in.

From great trochanter to outer condyle . . . . . . = 10¾ in.
Circumference at middle of thigh . = 12 in.
Tibia, from inner tuberosity to inner malleolus . . . . . = 9½ in.
Circumference of thickest part of leg . . . . . . = 11 in.
Circumference of leg just above ankle . . . . . . = 6 in.

Upper extremities.—The deltoid seems a little hypertrophied, but not so much as the glutæi. The triceps seems also somewhat hypertrophied. The pectorals and scapular muscles almost completely atrophied, and the latissimus dorsi can scarcely be felt. The head of the humerus can be felt with perfect ease, and can be partially dislocated and reduced, the ligaments being very lax; the bony points around the joint can be very easily felt. The biceps and coracobrachialis are also very much wasted. The muscles of the forearm and of the thumb and fingers are fairly developed, and of their natural size.

Measurements of upper extremities—
 From acromion to outer condyle .= $8\frac{1}{4}$ in.
 Circumference at middle of arm .= 6 in.
 Length of ulna . . . .= $7\frac{1}{4}$ in.
 Circumference of forearm just below
  condyles . . . . .= $6\frac{3}{4}$ in.

Trunk.—As before said, the lumbo-sacral curve is greatly exaggerated. The erector spinæ is immensely hypertrophied, and can be felt as a thick, hard mass on each side of the spine. The spinous processes of the vertebræ lie in a groove between these masses of muscle. In the space between the crest of the ilium and the last rib the thick hard edge of the erector spinæ can be felt distinctly. The belly is big, but the muscles forming its wall do not appear to be either wasted or hypertrophied. The cremasters act readily. The chest is broad and deep, and the costal angle exceedingly obtuse; its conical shape can be very distinctly seen, owing to the wasting of the pectorals. The serratus magnus is large, and its serrations can be seen with great clearness through the skin; it is not hard, like the erector spinæ, but appears to act naturally.

The action of the diaphragm in respiration was carefully watched, and found to be the same as in a healthy person. The intercostals appear to act fairly.

Measurements of chest—
  From acromion to acromion . = 10 in.
  Circumference just below axilla :
    On expiration . . . = 24 in.
    On inspiration . . . = $25\frac{1}{2}$ in.
  Circumference on a level with ensiform cartilage :
    On expiration . . . = 26 in.
    On inspiration . . . = $27\frac{1}{2}$ in.

Head and neck.—The sterno-mastoid is rather wasted. The depressors of the os hyoides are capable of fairly vigorous action. It is doubtful whether there is anything abnormal with the trapezius, and the other muscles of that group; if anything they are hypertrophied. His temporal muscles are undoubtedly hypertrophied, and, seen from the front, form a small tumour outside each orbit. His masseters seem somewhat increased in size, but this is difficult to ascertain. The facial muscles of expression appear sluggish in their action. His orbiculares are wasted; he can shut his eyes, but cannot screw them up tightly. He cannot frown, and can elevate his eyebrows but little. The muscles acting on the mouth do not seem defective at first sight, but on making him go through various grimaces, it is seen that he has not the command over the upper lip that he has over the lower; this, perhaps, is from misapprehension of directions. He puts out his tongue in a peculiar way, it always being concave, and he does not protrude it beyond his lips unless told to put it out further, when he makes an effort; but it is never convex from side to side. No affection of any ocular muscle.

General appearance, &c.—He is a dull, heavy-looking boy, with a stolid, but somewhat cunning expression of countenance. His face is very fat, especially about the lower part; complexion sallow and pasty; skin thick, superficial veins cannot be distinctly seen through it. His head is very large (circumference where the hat fits twenty-one inches); its shape is broad rather than long. Hair thick, brown, and straight. Forehead rather high. Eyes brown, pupils large, eyelashes long, eyebrows thick at outer part, thick towards the median line. Nose flat and broad, especially broad at the bridge; alæ nasi thin, nasal aperture large. Ears small, but well shaped, lobules not ill developed. Lips thick, upper lip thicker than lower, angles of mouth somewhat inclined downwards. Thyroid gland enlarged but not greatly. Voice natural, clear, low-pitched. Bones of extremities well shaped; epiphyses not unduly large.

Mental condition.—He is stupid or dull, but rather cunning. He is generally good tempered, but is often passionate, and at times very sulky; he appears to possess a strong will (he has probably been spoilt at home). He is not timid or bashful in any way. He smiles when spoken to, answers questions readily, and he takes any experiments tried upon him in very good part. He cannot read, but knows his letters. He has an appreciation of music, and amuses the other patients by his singing, whistling, &c.

Nervous system.—He sleeps well. Has no fits or cramps of any kind. Sight good, ophthalmoscopic appearance normal. Hearing, taste, and smell good. Sensation, both painful, tactile, and thermic, appears to be very good all over the body. It cannot be estimated with the compasses, because the boy, whether from laziness or any other motive, does not (or perhaps cannot) give consistent answers. The atrophied muscles do not respond at all to electricity. The gastrocnemii and hamstring muscles contract under it. The other hypertrophied muscles were not tested with it.

Digestion and appetite good. Bowels regular.

Urine.—Sp. gr. generally rather high; acid; no albumen, no sugar.

Respirations, 18 per minute, taken minutely; no cough or dyspnœa.

Heart.—Cardiac dulness. reaches above to third rib; on the right to an inch beyond the sternum; on the left to within half an inch of nipple; apex beat under fifth rib, one inch to right of nipple, 88 per minute. Impulse normal. Sounds sharp and clearly defined, somewhat exaggerated. No murmur or thrill of any kind.

Temperature, taken at different times, always normal.

Remarks.—This case, for the very careful

notes of which I am indebted to my clinical clerk, Mr. Herman, is a very typical example of the disease so well described by Dr. Duchenne in the 'Transactions' of this Society. By the aid of the harpoon I extracted specimens of the muscle from both gastrocnemii. When examined by the microscope, it was noticed that the transverse striation of the muscular fibre was very indistinct, that there was a great increase of connective-tissue elements, and that there were numerous fat-globules, but they were distinctly external to the sarcolemma. There was no fatty degeneration of the muscular structure.

The treatment has been dietetical with the daily use of the faradic current. No improvement, however, has resulted. I think the best name for such cases is pseudo-hypertrophic paralysis.

A CASE

OF

PSEUDO-HYPERTROPHIC PARALYSIS.

'Path. Soc. Trans.,' vol. xxi, 1870.

SAMUEL RICHARDSON, aged eleven, admitted into the London Hospital 22nd February, 1870. There is no family history of insanity, nor any mental affection. The father appears a man of average intelligence; the mother is certainly below the average. She appears a woman of a desponding, irresolute disposition, and of very slow perception; I should think her inclined to melancholia. She is thirty-seven, and has had six children; this one is the eldest. It was born at full time, after a tedious labour, lasting two days and a half, and was delivered with instruments. She has had one miscarriage, and one child, her fourth, died aged one year and a half, from "fits," which it had had from a month old; at the time it died it had not cut any of its teeth. All the rest are living. She states that while pregnant with this child she was in very delicate health, but she is unable to describe any definite ailment. She has always had plenty of food. The father is a mason, aged thirty-three; has always had good health. During the first two or three years of his marriage he used to be very frequently intoxicated. This child was two years old before he had any teeth, or before he could walk, and he was always very fretful. The mother says that while he was teething, and afterwards, he used to suffer from attacks of "inflammation," but I cannot make out what she means by this. She does not think that in intellectual capacity he is behind the other children. Five years ago he had rheumatic fever; was in bed six months, all his joints being affected. Previous to that was quite well. Since then has suffered at times with rheumatic pains in different joints, and has been weak and delicate. About twelve months ago his parents first noticed that when he walked he used to "bend his back in;" his stomach sticking out in front and his buttocks behind. About nine months ago it was first observed that when running, his legs would give way, and he would fall with his legs under him. About eight months ago he began to complain of his back hurting him. About this time, his mother says, he began to lose strength in his arms. His walking has since gradually got worse; he began to be unable to run before he was unable to walk. His falls became more and more frequent; at last he would fall down about every five or six yards. For the past two months he has been unable to walk without assistance, and for the past fortnight has been unable to walk at all. For some time past, his mother says, he has been losing flesh. She says he has lost flesh in his calves and buttocks as well as in other places.

He is rather small for his age. His height is 3 ft. $10\frac{1}{2}$ in. His aspect is that of a dull, backward child. He has a vacant, apathetic, timid expression of face. Complexion fair, cheeks fresh-coloured; hair brown, thick, straight, and fine; eyelashes long and fine; eyebrows thin, a wide interval between them in the middle line. Pupils large, irides dark, sclerotics of a bluish tint; eyeballs prominent. Nose broad, especially at the bridge, alæ nasi thick; nasal apertures large. Forehead high, round, protuberant; face fat, especially at lower part; lips thick, upper lip the thicker, and is broad and long. Bones well shaped; epiphyses not unduly large. Finger ends square. Costal angle acute. Palatal arch contracted; teeth crowded and irregular; skin thick, superficial veins can be seen, but not distinctly. Ears of moderate size, lobules small. Circumference of head where hat fits, $20\frac{1}{2}$ inches.

He cannot stand by himself. When told to try and stand by himself, he bends forward, and stands on tiptoe, but he cannot succeed. If he be held up by the arms there is a tendency to bend his body at the hips. If he be made to put his heels to the ground the tendency is greater. If left unsupported, his body bends forward at the hips, and he falls with his legs under him; but he can stand if support be given by the hand pressing his buttocks forward, though he does so in a tottering way. He can sit up without assistance, but he likes to have one hand behind him as a kind of prop. If he be laid down on his back, he cannot get up by himself without great exertion; he accomplishes it by turning on his side, and by pulling at the clothes brings his body to the proper angle with his legs, he then clutches at the bedclothes and pulls himself up by them.

His body is wasted, but not markedly so. The lumbo-sacral curve is slightly exaggerated; the glutæal region is larger and more rounded than is consistent with his wasted condition, and it is very hard. The erector spinæ is about as large as it should be for a boy of his age, but is much harder and firmer than it ought to be. The abdomen is large. It is difficult to estimate the size of the abdominal muscles, but they are capable of fairly vigorous action; (measurement around pelvis over most prominent part of glutæi, twenty-two inches; from one iliac spine to the other, eight inches). He moves his legs about badly, and without much power. If asked to cross his legs, he takes hold of one with his hands and lifts it over the other. He can perform this movement without the aid of his hands, but does so slowly, and with apparent exertion. As he lies on the bed, if told to draw up his legs, he does this with more force than he can any other movement. On sitting him on the edge of the bed he can raise his feet to a right angle with his body, *i. e.* extend his knees; but a 1 lb. weight attached to his great toe is sufficient to prevent him. On placing him on his face, he can flex his leg on the thigh, but a 2 lb. weight attached to his great toe prevents him. He can move his feet laterally at the ankle-joint, and does this pretty well. He can extend and flex his foot a little at the ankle, but he does not do this nearly so well as he should. He can move his toes but slightly.

On examining the muscles, the tensor vaginæ femoris is felt enlarged and very hard. The sartorius he can put in action, and it does not seem wasted. The quadriceps extensor seems harder than it should be, but this is difficult to estimate, as is the size of the muscle. The flexor muscles of the thigh are larger than ordinary. The adductors are small, but contract well when he puts them in action. The gastrocnemii are large and very hard; the extensor muscles and the peronei are also hard, and are certainly not wasted. The foot is in a state of talipes equino-varus: the tendo Achillis is very tense. The extensor brevis appears wasted, but it is difficult to tell. (*Measurements.*—From trochanter major to external condyle, $10\frac{3}{4}$ inches; from anterior superior spine of ilium to external condyle $12\frac{1}{4}$ in.: circumference at middle of thigh, $9\frac{1}{2}$ in.; length of tibia, from inner tuberosity to inner malleolus, $10\frac{1}{4}$ in.; circumference at thickest part of calf, $8\frac{5}{8}$ in.; just above ankle, $5\frac{3}{8}$ in.)

His chest is long and narrow; costal angle very acute. Breathing mostly abdominal. When told to take a deep breath, he does so with his diaphragm; the chest moves but slightly, and the intercostal spaces sink in. The serratus magnus can be felt, and appears about normal.

He can move his hands and arms in any direction, but has not much strength in them. He can take a 2 lb. weight and elevate it above his head, but no heavier weight. A boy aged nine, in the same ward, suffering from pulmonary disease, can lift 6 lb.; on resisting the action of the triceps with a 2 lb. weight, he can just extend his arm. As to the biceps, he cannot flex his arm against 2 lb., but he can against 1 lb. He can move his fingers readily, but has not much strength in them.

On examination of the muscles, the pectorals, biceps, and coraco-brachialis are most markedly wasted. The deltoid is hypertrophied, also the triceps, in a very noticeable manner. The latissimus dorsi is wasted, also the sterno-mastoid, very decidedly. The scapular muscles are hypertrophied, as is the trapezius. The muscles of the forearm and hand seem neither hypertrophied nor wasted. (*Measurements.*—Circumference of thorax: just below axillæ, on inspiration, $20\frac{1}{2}$ inches, on expiration, $20\frac{1}{4}$ in.; at level of ensiform cartilage, on inspiration, $23\frac{1}{2}$ in., on expiration, $22\frac{1}{2}$ in.; from acromion to acromion, 10 in.; from acromion to outer condyle, $8\frac{1}{4}$ in.; circumference at middle of upper arm, right, $5\frac{3}{4}$ in.; left $6\frac{1}{8}$ in.; length of ulna, $7\frac{1}{4}$ in.; circumference of thickest part of forearm, 6 in.; circumference of neck, $10\frac{1}{4}$ in.)

His facial muscles of expression appear sluggish in their action. He can screw his eyes up firmly, and can elevate his eyebrows; but I cannot get him to frown; whether he can or cannot I do not know. He seems to have but little power over his lips. His face seems remarkably devoid of expression; on trying to make him grimace, he either will not or cannot contort his face as told. When he laughs he does so in a feeble sort of way; I cannot make him laugh aloud, or put on a broad grin, but the other patients say that he does. His temporals and masseters seem normal. His thyroid gland does not seem enlarged. He puts his tongue out in a feeble manner; he puts it out slowly, and a very little distance, but he can put it out far if he likes.

Mentally he is certainly below the average of a boy of his age. He is very slow in his answers; seems afraid of everyone, and often cries. The men in the ward remark that the other boy (Round), although more paralysed, is "the best man of the two." He knows his letters, but cannot read. He can do very simple sums in arithmetic, such as that two and two make four, but three and four he says make eight. He is cunning, although stupid.

He sleeps well. Has no fits or cramps of any kinds. No paralysis of any ocular muscle. Fundus oculi normal. Hearing, taste, and smell good. Sensation of every kind, painful, tactile, thermic, and electric, seems unimpaired: he does not answer properly, so that it is impossible to estimate it for purposes of comparison. Induced electricity applied to muscles does not produce contraction.

Appetite and digestion good, bowels regular.

Urine.—Sp. gr. about 1020; acid, no deposit, no albumen, no sugar.

Pulse 96. Cardiac dulness extends above to third rib; on the right, to right margin of sternum; on the left, to half an inch beyond the nipple; below, to the sixth rib. Apex-beat under fifth rib, half an inch to the right of the nipple. The impulse is increased, but is not heaving, nor is there a thrill. The first sound is doubled, but there is no decided murmur.

Respirations 20 per minute. No cough, no dyspnœa. Temperature normal.

Remarks.—This case presents a very good example of pseudo-hypertrophic paralysis in an earlier condition than that of "Round," previously reported. I am again indebted to my clinical clerk, Mr. Herman, for the very careful notes of the case. I did not extract any specimens of muscle, in consequence of rather troublesome wounds having been produced in the previous case.

It is worthy of being noted that this is the seventh case of pseudo-hypertrophic paralysis which has come under my observation, and that in each case there has existed more or less mental feebleness.

The treatment has been dietetical, with the daily employment of faradisation. No perceptible improvement of any kind has been observed.

ON THE RELATION

OF THE

TEETH AND MOUTH TO MENTAL DEVELOPMENT.

'Trans. Odontological Soc.,' vol. iv, 1871-2.

Gentlemen,—When your President did me the honour of requesting me to read a paper before your Society, I felt at first some reluctance, from the consciousness that one of a very practical character was not within the scope of my power.

It occurred to me, however, that there was a branch of inquiry in which I felt considerable interest, and which had some slight bearing on the department of medical science represented by this Society. I thought, moreover, that I should derive great gain myself in bringing my observations before you, from the fact that while some of my work has been with a somewhat special class of humanity, you would be able to correct or confirm my views from observations over a wider and more varied field. It is thus, by the comparison of results obtained from opposite standpoints that broad principles may be elicited, where otherwise narrow, and possibly mistaken, views might be entertained.

At an early period of my study of the mental affections of childhood and youth, I became convinced that the question involved a far larger region of inquiry than the mere psychological phenomena which were presented before me,—that, interesting as were the examples of mental deviations which were the every-day object of one's contemplation, they were really only a part of the great subject; and one became convinced, from observation, that the physical deviations were as interesting and important as the psychical, in relation to the study of mental alienation, and especially to that form of it which had a congenital origin or proclivity. It became clear to me that idiocy and imbecility were not simply disturbances of brain-power,—were not simply nerve-lesions in the narrowed acceptation of the term,—but were profound diseases involving almost every organ and system of organs in the body. True, the encephalic ganglia were found altered, either in quality or quantity, or both; the convolutions of the brain might be reduced to quadrumanous simplicity in one case, or present remarkable symmetricality in another; but these were conditions that could only be ascertained on post-mortem inspection. The question that presented itself to me was,—Were there any outward and visible signs of inward mental disturbance? If idiocy were something more than brain alteration, it followed that an inquiry into the condition of the other organs might establish some correlative change in them. With this object in view, I made a careful investigation into the bodily condition of nearly a thousand feeble-minded youths—their height, weight, and bodily conformation; into the condition of their muscular development, the state of their eyes, the shape of their ears; and last, but not least, into the structure of their mouths and the contents of the oral cavity. It was in my inquiry into the condition of the teeth and mouth especially that I arrived at the conclusion that, in by far the larger number of instances, I was able to indicate the period at which the depressed condition commenced and to predicate in some degree the amount of improvement which physical, intellectual, and moral training might possibly effect.

Thus an examination of the mouth afforded me a valuable guide both as to diagnosis and prognosis in cases which, without such guide, would be surrounded with insurmountable difficulty.

In consultations one is often pressed by the friends of the patient for an opinion as to the date at which the affection commenced. It is always a relief if an opinion can be given that the child was born intelligent; that the calamity is the result of some after-birth catastrophe. Curiously enough, there is often a degree of wounded pride if it is decided that the child was defective from birth. It is by an appeal to the physical conformation only that the decision can be justly made. In children whose idiocy is accidental, arising from causes operating after uterine life, there is but slight deviation from normal condition in the state of the mouth and teeth while it is in those whose malady is congenital, especially where arising from causes operating at a very early period of embryonic life, that the deviation of the mouth and its appendages from the normal condition is most pronounced.

It often happens to me to see children, about whom the only anxiety is that they do not speak. The parents seek for an explanation in the condition of the palate, little suspecting that the palatal deformity is only one of the manifestations of a congenital mental defect, in which ideas are so little formulated that language is not needed.

I could occupy a large portion of the time of this meeting in illustrating the value of an appeal to the condition of the mouth as an aid to diagnosis in such cases; a few cases must suffice.

A year or two since a very intelligent medical practitioner in the country was called in to treat a case of infantile convulsions. The condition of the child was desperate. He poured from an ewer a stream of cold water over the occiput of the child; the convulsions ceased, the patient was rescued from impending death, but grew up to be an idiot. The friends of the child took up a position which involved a trial in a court of law, equivalent to an action for malpraxis against the medical man. By a judge's order, I, with other medical men, saw the child; and we were able to say not only that the child was an idiot then, but, by an examination of the mouth, to assert that the idiocy was embryonic as to date, that the convulsion was an epiphenomenon, and that the medical man was in no way responsible for the mental condition of the child whose life he had rescued. Thus, by an appeal to physical conformation, we were able to date the mental defect, and to save the reputation of a medical brother from undeserved opprobrium.

It will be within your remembrance that this town was some years since greatly moved by a sensational trial before a Master in Lunacy, in which an attempt was made to save from himself a youth with an honoured name. "Liberty of the Subject" was the popular cry, and after conflicting evidence, the popular will prevailed, and the free agent went rapidly to his doom. The counsel for the defence, in specious terms suggested that the mistake about this young man's imbecility arose from a defect in his mouth, from which imperfect speech resulted. I showed at that time—too late, however, to influence the verdict—that that was the most important admission that could be made,—that, given any amount of mental obliquity, no stronger confirmatory proof could have been adduced of his imbecility than the physical defects of mouth to which this lisping speech was due. The sequel proved the true nature of the case.

No less valuable, however, is a study of the condition of the mouth as a means of prognosis in any given case. In children who exhibit any want of mental power, or present anomalous moral or intellectual symptoms, no more anxious question is suggested than that relating to their probable future. The disposition of property, and other family arrangements, depend a good deal on the answer which is given. We have learned by experience this important fact, that the child who has been born with defective intellect is more susceptible of improvement by physical and intellectual training than the child who has been born with full possession of his brain-power, and has afterwards lost it. It follows, that of two children who are the subjects of solicitude, other things being equal, there is greater probability of improvement for the patient with an ill-developed, than the one with a damaged brain. Often it happens that a microcephalic idiot, about whom the inexperienced would entertain no sort of hope, will far outshine, under intellectual training, the fine, well-developed boy the membranes of whose brain have been the subject of inflammatory lesion, and about whose capillaries lymph has been inextricably effused. An appeal to the condition of the mouth is an important aid in determining whether the lesion on which the mental weakness depends is of intra-uterine or of post-uterine origin. In the event of the mouth being abnormal, it indicates a congenital origin; while if the mouth be well formed, and the teeth in a healthy condition, it would lead to the opinion that the calamity had occurred subsequently to embryonic life.

Of course, our judgment would be formed after a physical examination of every organ—of the condition of the ears and eyes—of the shape of the cranium; but what I want to enforce is, that most important information is derived from an examination of the mouth.

I have had this day brought to me a young girl of manifestly defective power, and the parents were extremely anxious to know whether it was a congenital case. Their anxiety was based partly on an unwillingness for either branch of the family to allow that there was on their side any hereditary tendency to mental disease—a sort of rivalry as to the purity of the two antecedent sources; but mainly also to ascertain with what degree of fear they must watch the development of their other children, and how it might affect the education of their sons, or the marriage prospects of their daughters. No study of the mental phenomena themselves would have enabled me to venture an opinion; but an examination into the totality of the physical conformation in general, and of the mouth in particular, enabled me to refer the calamity, with a considerable degree of certainty, to an accidental cause, probably a sunstroke in the tropics; to clear the other members of the family from the suspicion of insane proclivity, and to defend the purity of the rival stocks.

Let us now consider what are the conditions of the mouth associated with mental defect.

The lips are usually thick, the thickness being greatly more marked in the lower than in the upper one. In addition to the thickening, they are often striated, marked by transverse fissures; this character is more generally seen in a class of congenital idiots, which I have elsewhere described as Mongolian idiots, from their resemblance in physical character to the Mongolian race. Often the lips are deficient in muscular power, which interferes with their prehensile function, and which also induces a tendency for the saliva to run over the chin. The mucous membrane is extremely liable to chronic inflammation, and ulceration is induced by the slightest pressure against prominent or uneven teeth. The glands of the mucous membrane of the mouth generally, as well as the salivary glands, are usually hypertrophied; and this is another factor in the production of stammering.

There is a marked postponement in the evolution of the first teeth. Looking over my notes of a very large number of cases, I find that the first dentition is almost invariably postponed. The ease with which dentition is effected varies; sometimes the teeth are cut so easily that no disturbance of the general health is observed;

in others it is the period at which violent convulsive attacks are developed, imperilling greatly the feeble mental endowment of the child. Contrary to the law that tissues which are slowly formed are the most persistent, these primary teeth have a more temporary existence than usual. They are frequently dark, speedily become carious, and their stunted growth often aggravated by the incessant grinding of the teeth, which is so frequent during the infantile life of such children. I have been curious to ascertain the cause of this grinding. In most cases it appears to be a kind of automatic movement, not depending on the direct influence of the will; one of those rhythmic movements of which there are several amongst children of this class. In others it would appear to be purposely developed to produce a monotonous sound, which imparts pleasure to the feeble-minded. Not only, however, are the primary teeth ill developed; they are often irregularly developed as to sequence. Nothing but disorder is noticed in their succession.

Just as the evolution of the temporary teeth is accompanied by cataclysmic effects, like phenomena not unfrequently accompany the evolution of the permanent teeth. The epileptiform convulsions which accompany the first, not unfrequently after a long interlude, reappear at the cutting of the second, to be followed by another interlude, and a recurrence at puberty. I have now under my observation a boy whose first teething was marked by paroxysmal phenomena of the most violent kind, which ceased when the physiological effort was over. He has now arrived at the period of second dentition, and the evolution of every tooth is accompanied by well-marked epileptic attacks and by a corresponding decadence in his stunted mental development.

The evolution of the second teeth is also frequently postponed, and there is slight irregularity in the sequence of their development. A marked character of the teeth is their irregularity as to position. They are often crowded— so crowded as to present their sides instead of their anterior surfaces. They are often arranged on different planes. The canine teeth are frequently unduly prominent, and a marked sulcus is sometimes seen between the incisors and canines, with prominence of the incisors. The teeth themselves present very frequently a honeycombed appearance, from an absence of continuity in the enamel, and they undergo speedy decay. Nothing is more marked than the temporary nature of the so-called permanent teeth.

It has been a matter of considerable interest to me to ascertain how frequently the syphilitic teeth, so well described by my friend and colleague Mr. Hutchinson, were to be met with among the feeble-minded; but the result of my inquiry has been to discover very few among them who were in this way indicated to be the subjects of congenital syphilis. Very few have had syphilitic teeth; but where I did discover them, I always had confirmatory evidence of the syphilitic history of the case, and the condition of the teeth was always associated with the chronic inflammation of the cornea to which Mr. Hutchinson has called attention. I have therefore been led to the conclusion that syphilis is not by any means an important factor in the production of congenital mental disease. The honeycombed teeth are, I am persuaded, perfectly distinct from the syphilitic, and are manifestations of that grave perversion of nutrition which implicates, in these cases, every tissue in the body.

The tongue presents peculiarities worthy of notice. It is frequently unusually large. Its inordinate size generally arises from increase in length, and also from an absence of muscular tonicity. The surface is often curiously corrugated, presenting numerous fissures. The surface is rendered still more rough from hypertrophy of the papillæ. Not only is the tongue inconveniently large, it is but feebly under the influence of the will. There is a want of co-ordination in its muscles; so that not only is the more intelligential act of speaking performed awkwardly even when there are ideas to be communicated, but the simple voluntary act of conveying the food to the posterior part of the mouth, where the reflex act of deglutition is excited, is effected with difficulty, and thus an almost instinctive act is rendered to some extent abortive.

Of most significant value, however, is the condition of the palate. I have made a very large number of careful measurements of the mouths of the congenitally feeble-minded and of intelligent persons of the same age, with the result of indicating, with some few exceptions, a markedly-diminished width between the posterior bicuspids of the two sides. The exceptions were some few cases of macrocephalic idiots, who had inordinately large crania, depending in some cases on hypertrophy of the brain, or more frequently on chronic hydrocephalus. In these exceptional cases the palates were as widely in excess, as in others they are less than the normal width. One result, or rather one accompaniment, of this narrowing is the inordinate vaulting of the palate, which assumes a roof-like form. The vaulting is not simply apparent from the approximation of the teeth of the two sides, it is absolute—the line of junction between the palatal bones occupying a higher plane. Often there is an antero-posterior sulcus corresponding to the line of approximation of the two bones.

There is very frequently a deficiency in the posterior part of the hard palate, from a want of development of the palatal process of the maxillary bone, as well as absence of the palatal process of the palate bone. As a result of this defect, the false palate hangs down abnormally, and interferes with clear phonation. At an early period of my investigations I was prepared to find a large number of cases of cleft palate. This does not appear, however, to be a frequent defect—not more, according to my statistics, than 5 in 1000 cases. Bisection of the uvula occurred 4 times in 1000, and absence of the uvula twice. The cause of the frequent excessive vaulting of the palate is not quite clear; it may possibly arise, as has been suggested, from arrest of development of the sphenoid bone, or defective growth of the bone. It has been attributed by one writer to a cause which I think cannot be allowed, viz. sucking the thumb. This gentleman attributes idiocy entirely, or almost entirely, to "fruitless sucking." The chain of events, according to his theory, is this:—The fruitless sucking gives rise to secretion of gastric juice in the stomach when it has no physiological use,—that this acts as an irritant on the intestinal mucous membrane, giving rise to diarrhœa and disturbed nutrition, eventuating in convulsions and idiocy; and that the roofed palate I have described is the physical result of the pressure of the child's thumb against the palate. Banish fruitless sucking, he says, and idiocy would be unknown. I believe this to be a thoroughly mistaken notion. Idiots are not much more prone to fruitless sucking than other children, and I have examined the palates of several fruitless suckers among the sane without finding the palatal defects I have described. I think it will require no argument to prove that the defects I have referred to are developmental defects, and that they betoken a cause long anterior to the time when sucking the thumb is practised, unless that habit be an intra-uterine one. The theory overlooks the whole bearing of hereditary influence, and of nervous shocks and physical illness to the pregnant woman, as potent causes of imbecility in the offspring, and negatives the idea of the congenital nature of the ailment.

There is one practical point with reference to the palatal defect which has some interest to me. One of the greatest difficulties we have, but one which, when overcome, brings the greatest *kudos*, is the teaching an idiot or imbecile to speak. We have to furnish him with a vocabulary, to practise him in tongue gymnastics, to build up for him a language, and to lessen the mutiny of the muscles of his tongue. When all this is in part accomplished, the arched roof of the palate is a great trouble. Imperfect speech still remains. Can nothing be done mechanically in this direction? Can the members of this Society tell us of any success they have had by diminishing the palatal cavity among the sane that may augur hope for us with the insane? Often cases are met with where the palatal difficulty is just *the* hindrance to an improved imbecile mixing with the world, and taking his place with his fellows.

Among idiots and imbeciles there is often discovered a want of symmetry in the cranium. The plan which I adopt of taking the shape with a strip of lead shows this defect admirably, and enables me to sketch the precise deformity on paper. This want of symmetry also affects the bones of the jaw, leading to a great difference between the two halves of the maxillary bones. A very marked example of this kind was seen with me a short time since by my friend Mr. Ramsay, who advised the removal of some teeth to make room for the movements of the tongue. It was an excellent example also of the obtuseness to pain which is common among the feeble-minded. Often they are anxious to have their teeth extracted, as if it were a personal favour; they are flattered by the attention,—rarely do they care for the pain which is inflicted,—chloroform is for them a superfluity.

A want of symmetry is occasionally noticed in the palate when there is no very marked absence of symmetry elsewhere.

I might also mention anomalies of the tonsils and of the fauces, but these would have but little interest to you.

The gums are extremely prone to recede from the teeth, and to become tumid, as in the scorbutic condition.

The masticatory process is always performed with difficulty. The carious condition of the teeth is one cause of this, but it is principally due to the imperfection with which any voluntary act is performed. The sense of taste is obtuse, no medicine, however nauseous, is refused, and without care many will eat with indifference the most offensive garbage.

To sum up, we have in the condition of the mouths of idiots important data for distinguishing between idiocy of a congenital and that of a non-congenital origin, and to base thereon a prognosis as to relative improvement by treatment. They are, the thickness of the lower lip, the delay of dentition, premature caries of the teeth, the irregularity of dentition, the chronic inflammation of the gums and buccal mucous membrane; the height, angularity, and want of symmetry of the palatal vault; the long, corrugated, and coarsely-papulated tongue, and the hyper-secretion of saliva. Common to the congenital and non-congenital cases we meet with defect of mastication, a want of co-ordination of the muscles of the tongue, and the slight development of the faculty of speech.

I am anxious to hear from the members of this Society their own experience with regard to any feeble-minded patients that may have come under their observation, and how far the picture I have drawn from nature contrasts with what they meet with in members of a sane community. It is quite possible that some of the characters I have noted may be met with sometimes among those who are doing their work in the world, and are among the bread-winners of society. My own experience leads me to consider that they are exceptional cases. May not palatal deformities be indicative of a slightly degenerative process?

When investigating cretinism in the valleys of Piedmont, one is struck with the very gradual deterioration of the race. Some of the typical features of cretinism are met with among the grandparents, and we have been able to trace the increased degenerative stages through the children to the effete grandchildren.

I have often had a wish to measure and note the condition of the mouths of some of the progenitors of my patients, and trace—as I believe in some instances one could trace—the gradual deterioration of the species till it culminated in congenital imbecility.

That is just the link that I have not been able to forge. I know no men more likely than those I have the honour to address to-night, to be able to fill up, from their experience, the shortcomings of my own.

THE

OBSTETRICAL ASPECTS OF IDIOCY.

'Trans. Obstet. Soc.,' 1876.

IF one regards the large number of children in our community who grow up with defective mental power, children who, although not all fairly to be ranked among decided idiots, yet have such lesion of the faculties of perception and reasoning as to bring them under the category of the feeble-minded, and if one has reference to the terrible anxieties such children entail on their parents, and the burden they often are to the struggling members of our race, one cannot fail to be impressed with the importance of anything connected with the circumstances of such a condition.

I had therefore no difficulty in responding to an invitation to bring before this Society some of the opinions which have been impressed upon me, having relation to facts which come under the immediate regard of gentlemen practising the obstetrical branch of our profession.

The data on which these remarks are based have been collected over a space of more than eighteen years, and relate to two thousand children who during that time have come under my observation, and about whom I have been able to gather information. They have been collected with great care and with an anxious desire to exclude all doubtful matter.

One very interesting and important point suggested by my inquiries is that of primogeniture. We know how much our political system hangs on the laws of primogeniture, how the first-born inherits property and inherits too the power to rule over his fellows, and how much our whole social structure is built thereon. Nevertheless, the result of my statistics shows that no less than 24 per cent. of all the idiot children I have seen are primiparous offspring. How many primiparæ there are who, although not coming under the category of idiots are yet somewhat incapable, my statistics, of course, do not reveal.

It will be obvious, however, that before any real value can be assigned to this statement it will be necessary to inquire into the average number of children belonging to these families. This I have been at great pains to ascertain, and I find that up to the time I had been consulted in each case 6·91, or nearly seven, was the average number of living children born to the parents who have had an idiot child. Fourteen per cent. were second born, 9 per cent. fourth, 5 per cent. fifth, 7 per cent. sixth, 10 per cent. seventh, 2 per cent. eighth, 9 per cent. ninth, 2 per cent. tenth, 2 per cent. eleventh, 1 per cent. twelfth, 3 per cent. thirteenth, and 1 per cent. fourteenth. The question naturally presents itself as to what should give this undue preponderance of idiocy to primiparæ. I have no doubt that it may be largely attributed to the exalted emotional life of the mother; her life is one of exaggerated hopes and fears; she is prone to live in an unnaturally expectant atmosphere. She is going through an experience altogether new, with untried responsibilities both social and domestic. She is more than usually responsive to external impressions and influences, certainly more to subjective feelings and whims. But, as I have elsewhere observed, it would betoken a narrow view of the matter if we restricted our attention to the emotional life of the mother and kept out of sight the emotional tendencies of the father. No one who has seen much of private practice is unaware how much men are frequently influenced by the responsibilities of the matrimonial state, how the doubts as to their own virility, of their being able to make a position in the world after having given hostages to fortune, the disturbing elements of a new social position both with regard to their immediate circle of friends and to the new relationships formed. All these and some others are perturbing influences to many men, and while, therefore, the emotional life of the incubating mother is an important element, the emotional tendencies of the procreating father must be regarded too as a cause of the increased frequency of primiparous idiots.

But there is another cause which will naturally occur to the Fellows of this Society as obstetricians. I refer to the increased difficulties of parturition. No one can have regard to the smallness of the maternal passages, to their undilated character, to the rigidity of the perinæum, and to the tediousness of the labour, without being impressed with the influence they must have in interfering with the integrity of the cranial contents, and to their inducing a condition perilous to the future mental health of the little one. They are conditions which frequently give rise to instrumental interference, but above all to a state of suspended animation which in my opinion it should be the earnest desire of the obstetrician to avoid.

I think it cannot fail to strike the Fellows of the Society as a very important fact that no fewer than 20 per cent. of the idiots of my investigation were born with well-marked symptoms of suspended animation — symptoms which required judicious and strenuous efforts to overcome in order to effect resuscitation. Moreover, it is specially interesting that while, as we have said, 24 per cent. of idiots generally are primiparous, as many as 40 per cent. of resuscitated idiots come under this category. Clearly, then, suspended animation is a condition as far as possible to be avoided by the practical obstetrician.

Bearing on this part of the subject is the question of instrumental interference. I have made a careful inquiry on this subject over a very large area, and with the expectation I should find a large amount of idiocy to be the result of "meddlesome midwifery," but I am bound to say that my statistics falsify my anticipations, and redound to the care with which instruments are employed in parturition. I find from an examination of all my cases about which positive information could be obtained that in only 3 per cent. were the forceps employed. In every case, however, where they had been employed the friends of the child believed that the instrument alone was the cause of the disaster, while in nearly every case I could discover quite sufficient to account for the mental defect in the neurotic history of the progenitors. In a very few cases, only a small fractional percentage, could I arrive at the conclusion that the use of the forceps was the principal cause of the calamity.

I find in a very large number of my cases that the labour was stated to be unusually tedious and prolonged. Dr. Playfair has shown that the employment of the forceps does not interfere with the viability of the offspring, and that a prolonged labour is more compromising to the life-prospects of the child than a judicious and timely application of the forceps. Certainly my statistics make clear to me, contrary to what some years since was advanced by Dr. Arthur Mitchell, and in harmony with Dr. Ramsbotham's experience, that the use of the forceps is not an important factor in the production of brain disease. When, however, it is borne in mind how frequent is the association of suspended animation with idiocy, it cannot, I think, be too strongly enforced that the mental integrity of the child is more likely to be compromised by a prolonged pressure in the maternal passages than by skilled employment of artificial assistance. The accoucheur who postpones instrumental help often does so at the risk of terrible consequences to the nervous system of the little one he is solicitous to protect.

I have collected a good deal of information as to the influence of twin births. There is a general prejudice that the individuals of twin births are not strong physically. Mr. Galton has been collecting materials on this and cognate subjects, but I am not aware of his results. Taking my last thousand cases, only 2 per cent. were twins, while, singularly enough, the same thousand show that in 2 per cent. of the cases the mothers had given birth to twins who were not afflicted in any way. This would appear to indicate that the existence of twins does exercise some prejudicial influence, seeing that among one thousand mothers who have borne an idiot child, where they have happened to be twins, no fewer than a quarter of them were idiots.

A very potential cause in the production of idiocy is the physical health of the mother during gestation. In 20 per cent. of my cases there was a history of marked physical disturbance. In 4 per cent. there was a history of serious falls—falls which were followed by alarming uterine hæmorrhage. In 6 per cent. there was an account of prolonged ill health, and in no fewer than 10 per cent. was there a history of sickness—cases in which the vomiting had been marked and persistent, and had given rise to anxiety on account thereof. I feel quite sure that sickness during pregnancy is an important producer of idiocy and is a symptom which, from this grave aspect of it, claims the earliest attention of the obstetrician. It will be readily understood that any cause which would render the mother anæmic would be a source of peril to the mental health of the child.

From what I have already said it will have been gathered that I lay great stress on the emotional life of the child-bearing woman as a potential cause of idiocy. I cannot, however, attach greater importance to this aspect of the subject than it deserves. It is one of most serious importance and bespeaks one's careful regard. In no fewer than in 32 per cent. of my cases was there a well-founded history of great physical disturbance in the mother by fright, intense anxiety, or great emotional excitement. They were all cases in which a strong impression had been made on the mind. In a large number of instances the fright was attended by syncope. They were cases of fright arising from threatened outrage to the person, or where they had seen their own children in great peril or killed, or where intense anxiety had existed in consequence of the fatal illness of their husband or the loss of several of their children. No doubt they were troubles in many cases which might have been borne with equanimity by a philosopher, but the mothers possibly were more than usually responsive, and with an unstable equilibrium required only the stimulus of fear or anxiety to exercise a morbid influence on the development of their children. No doubt the emotional tendency of the mother, as depending on the same neurosis, may be regarded as a cause, but the actively potential cause in all the cases I have referred to was mainly the undue response to some external impression. The lesson to be gathered from such data is a very important one, viz. to maintain the child-bearing woman in the most equable state, to shield her as much as possible from all causes which would disturb unduly her emotional life, and to maintain in her that hopeful spirit and placid calm which is so much to be desired both for the woman herself as well as for the infant she is incubating. These data teach us how important it is that for women generally the emotions should not be cultivated at the sacrifice of their judgment and self-control.

The relation of sex to idiocy presents some matters of interest; there is a marked preponderance in the number of male over female idiots. The proportion among the two thousand I have noted stands in the ratio of 2·1 to ·9, or rather more than twice as many male as female. It is, I think, a very fair conclusion to arrive at that one very important factor is the increased dimension of the male over the female infantile cranium. This would be likely to give rise to prolonged and difficult parturition, to that continued pressure and that suspended animation which I regard as so disastrous to the cerebral functions. Another reason is the greater tendency, according to my notes, to infantile convulsions among males who have become idiots than among females who have become idiots, a circumstance which gives rise to a larger amount of what I call *accidental* idiocy among males. These statistics are, moreover, in harmony with what we know of the greater viability of female over male children. The question of sex opens up many interesting problems in relation to idiocy. I can only here intimate that where the origin is purely of a neurotic character my notes show that when the neurosis is paternal the male progeny are liable to suffer and the female to escape; where, on the contrary, the neurosis is maternal the female progeny are likely to bear the stress.

I have been at some pains to ascertain whether there is any relation between the administration of ergot of rye and idiocy. I have found, however, the answers so vague and the knowledge of my informants so uncertain that it has proved quite hopeless to arrive at any results which would have a scientific basis. Often the mothers have imagined that ergot had been used when there had been no such administration, and it is obvious that in many cases the medicine may have been taken without the mother being conscious that any drug had been made use of.

The diagnosis and prognosis of idiocy are both matters which perforce fall to the lot of the obstetrician, and it is of no small importance that he should have definite bases on which to form and give an opinion. An error in diagnosis would lead in all probability to unpleasant lessening of professional confidence.

The earliest observations, on the part of those in attendance on the child, of defect of sight, of unusual fretfulness or peculiarity as to taking food, should lead to very careful investigation of the structural formation of the child.

In cases which have a *congenital origin* you may find very early physical signs of serious trouble. The cranium must be examined as to its configuration, giving special heed to want of symmetry, to extreme dolicocephalism, to extreme brachycephalism, to rapid shelving at the occipital region, to the condition of the sutures, their premature or deferred synostosis, and especially to the frontal region which often displays the mediofrontal suture still existing, whereas there should have been complete coalescence of the two halves of the frontal bone during intrauterine life.

Examination of the ocular media and retina will remove the notion of blindness, and indicate that the defect in taking notice of external objects is rather one of cerebral than optical defect. The presence of strabismus should be noted, and the integument about the eye should be examined especially for semilunar folds of skin at the inner canthus—folds which are more frequently present in feeble-minded children than in others, and which I have been accustomed to describe as epicanthic folds. They are according to my experience marks of developmental degeneracy, and should be looked for. The position of the eyes is worthy of note, whether the inner canthi are too nearly approximated, as met with in microcephalic or scaphocephalic idiots, or too widely separated, as obtains in macrocephalic and hydrocephalic idiots. Observation should also be made as to any oblique position of the eyes as well as their wide separation, such as is met with in that ethnical variety which I have elsewhere described as Mongolian idiocy, a variety of great clinical as well as biological interest, showing that degenerative causes may and often do remove children into a different ethnic type from that of their progenitors. Particular observation should be made as to that peculiar oscillation of the balls called nystagmus, which is very frequently met with in children of the feeble-minded class.

The appearance of the external ear should be noticed, the condition of the pinna, the absence of a helix, and whether the lobule be absent. Observation should also be made as to the seat of implantation of the ear, which in idiots is usually placed further back in relation to the head and face than in normal children. No feature is more worthy of regard than the configuration and position of the external ear.

The mouth should be examined as to its palate, whether it be arched or Gothic-shaped; the tongue, whether it be too large, rugous, fissured, and with its papillæ enlarged; the jaw, as to the angle formed by the ascending and horizontal rami, which in idiots is more obtuse than usual.

Examination should be made of the surface of the body as to the condition of the skin—noting whether it has a lax and soddened appearance, especially on the extremities, and whether there be any defective coalescence at the bottom of the spine. The muscular system should be examined, special observation being made as to the existence of any automatic movements, contractures, or spastic rigidity. In early childhood as well as in more advanced life too much attention cannot be given to these physical signs of cerebral disease. They are, many of them, the marks of that kind of idiocy which is inherited or congenital in its origin, of that kind which is so often met with as the outcome of a gradually degenerating race.

Idiocy, however, is not always strictly *congenital;* in a large number of cases it is acquired or *accidental.* This includes those cases which occur from inflammation, often of a slow and insidious character, of the meninges whereby products are thrown out which afterwards interfere with the nutritive supply to the encephalon. It includes also the recoveries, although very rare, from tubercular meningitis, from infantile convulsions, and from acute diseases of various kinds, also those arising from traumatic injury as well as those where narcotics have been injudiciously and probably furtively given.

It is of great importance to be able to differentiate these accidental cases from the congenital ones, and this can only be done by having regard to the physical diagnosis I have before referred to. Often the friends of the children refer the origin of the disaster to a careless nurse who has let the child fall, to some remembered fright, or to an accoucheur who has used instruments unadvisedly ; but a reference to the physical condition of the child may tell one that the cause was long antecedent to the one suggested, and that far back in intra-uterine life, or possibly before, in the history of the progenitors, must the real cause be traced.

Not only is physical examination important in a diagnostic point of view; it is of no less value, as we shall see, in prognosis. What is to be the future of our child? is a question which will be put with more or less earnestness, usually with an earnestness from which there is no escape, and the reply will be treasured for years to come. I find that a large number of replies are given, apparently based on some sort of belief in periodic leaps. The favourite epoch is seven years. The friends are often lulled into a false security under the notion that at seven, fourteen, or twenty-one years of age all will come right. I know nothing of such cataclysmal improvements. The misfortune is that such opinions prevent all active means being employed, and when the longed-for time arrives it is found that precious opportunities have been lost, that with increased physical development there has come a stronger will, more resolute disobedience, and an absence of intellectual and moral growth which proper training might have effected.

But a no less fallacious opinion is often based on the good looks of the patient. The child probably does not speak at the proper time, rolls its head in a rhythmical way, looks into space, or makes monotonous noises with its lips. "Oh!" it is often said, "have no anxiety, all will come right; he is so bright-looking, so comely, he has no deformity of head, no lesion of limb." The friends have no difficulty in falling in with such a doctrine, and they await in full reliance the future which is predicated, but it is a future which never comes. It is experience alone that tells one that the prognosis in such a case is far less hopeful than in the case of one whose misplaced eyes, ill-shaped cranium, and distorted face gives ready indication of his feeble mind.

The case we have been considering is one of *accidental* origin. Something since birth has given rise to the disaster and has left no trace on his exterior. With such an one we are able to predict much less response to training than in the case of one whose defects have had an origin anterior to birth. It may be taken as a rule which has but few exceptions, that congenital idiocy is more amenable to training than post-congenital, that, in fact, it is more hopeful to have to do with an ill-developed than with a damaged brain, and having regard to what I have laid down as to the physical signs and configuration of congenital idiocy, that the prognosis is, contrary to what is so often thought, inversely as the child is comely, fair to look upon, and winsome.

It will be readily conceived how many interesting points of departure are suggested by the topics I have touched on. I have endeavoured, however, not to wander into simply philosophical paths, but to confine myself to what I considered had most direct bearing on " the obstetrical aspect of idiocy."

www.ingramcontent.com/pod-product-compliance
Lightning Source LLC
Chambersburg PA
CBHW022043230426
43672CB00008B/1058